# Your Dog

In real life Elizabeth Charles is the veterinary surgeon Pamela Tinslay. She qualified at the Royal Veterinary College, London, before emigrating to Australia in 1954 and now runs a veterinary practice in Sydney. For many years, under the name of Kate Newby, she wrote 'Pet Vet' for the Sydney *Sun* and had her own talk-back programme for Radio 2GB. She is the author of the enormously successful book *Animal Doctor*. For over 30 years her articles have been published in *Woman's Day*.

Jim Fraser is a dog trainer specialising in behaviour problems. He is consultant trainer for the Guide Dogs' 'Pets as Therapy' programme and animal behaviourist of the RSPCA in New South Wales.

*For Dawn and Stefanie*
*and my daughters Sally and Tabitha*

# Your Dog

A practical Australian guide to behaviour and training

**ELIZABETH CHARLES**
**with Jim Fraser**

VIKING O'NEIL

Acknowledgements: The author and publishers gratefully acknowledge the assistance of Petcare Information Advisory Service for supplying the colour photographs. The author would also like to thank Dorothy Rich for her support and help in reading the manuscript.

Viking O'Neil
Penguin Books Australia Ltd
487 Maroondah Highway, PO Box 257
Ringwood, Victoria 3134, Australia
Penguin Books Ltd
Harmondsworth, Middlesex, England
Viking Penguin, A Division of Penguin Books USA Inc.
375 Hudson Street, New York, New York 10014, USA
Penguin Books Canada Limited
10 Alcorn Avenue, Toronto, Ontario, Canada M4V 3B2
Penguin Books (N.Z.) Ltd
182–190 Wairau Road, Auckland 10, New Zealand

First published by Penguin Books Australia Ltd 1993

10 9 8 7 6 5 4 3 2 1

Copyright © Elizabeth Charles, 1993

Produced by Viking O'Neil
56 Claremont Street, South Yarra, Victoria 3141, Australia
A Division of Penguin Books Australia Ltd

Typeset in Cheltenham Light by Midland Typesetters, Maryborough, Victoria
Design by Meredith Parslow
Illustrations by Steve Panozzo
Black and white photographs by Bruce Postle
Printed in Australia by Griffin Paperbacks, Adelaide

National Library of Australia
Cataloguing-in-Publication data

Charles, Elizabeth, 1928–
  Your dog.

  Includes index.
  ISBN 0 670 90529 1.

  1. Dogs. 2. Dog breeds – Australia. I. Fraser, Jim, 1948–   . II.
  Title.

636.7

# Contents

**Preface**                                                              ix

## Part I   Choosing Your Dog

1  **So you think you want a dog?**                                       3
Fitting in: dogs and their owners • Why own a dog? all the wrong
reasons • The dog owner in the modern world: pros and cons

2  **Pitfalls of purchasing a pup and how to prevent them**             11
'My-other-dog' syndrome • A healthy pup: the signs • Decisions,
decisions ... • Costs and care • 'Where did you get that dog?':
sources • Crossbreeds and pedigree dogs • Selecting a pedigree
dog • Buying a pedigree pup • Visiting the breeder • Selecting
from the litter • The puppy test

3  **A handy guide to the breeds**                                       27
Don't judge a pooch by its cover: pedigree dogs • The toys • The
terriers • The gun dogs • The hounds • The working dogs
• The utility dogs • The non-sporting dogs

## Part II    Settling In

**4    Puppy comes home**                                                    **75**
Travel arrangements: the journey home • Arriving home • Sleeping arrangements: inside or out? • House-training • Playtime • Rest: for dog and owner • Loneliness: parting is such sweet sorrow • A good relationship: the perfect owner

**5    Nutrition and diet**                                                    **87**
Canine cuisine: what and how much? • It's in the can: a few questions answered • Diet: alternatives and additions

**6    How to survive the first four months**                              **97**
Patience is a prerequisite • The mind of a 6-week-old pup • Training a 6-week-old pup • Taking the lead • The big bad world outside • Recall work • Chaos while you're out: prevention • Discipline: a few rules for the owner • Playtime: not all fun and games

**7    How to survive your pup aged 4–6 months**                        **105**
The 'teenage' period • 'Don't invade my space': critical distance • Early training: 'do-it-yourself'

## Part III    Health Care

**8    First visit to the vet**                                              **111**
Bribery and blackmail: a two-way game

**9    Vaccinations**                                                        **114**
Diseases for which there are vaccinations

**10    Puppy care**                                                        **120**
Brushing and bathing • Pedicure • Ear care • Tooth care • Eye care • Dosing your dog • Cosmetic surgery

**11    Parasites**                                                          **133**
Internal parasites: worms • External parasites: fleas, ticks, mange and ringworm

## Part IV   Some Big Issues Tackled

**12   Your dog and the law: insurance**          **153**
'I'll see your dog in court' • Identification: dog tags and microchips

**13   Desex or not desex?: a difficult question**          **157**
Desexing the female: some questions answered • Desexing the male: male aggression and ego • Some fallacies and facts of life: love and sex

**14   Body language: understanding dogspeak**          **165**
A vocabulary of dogspeak

**15   Training**          **172**
Why bother? • Training methods

**Epilogue**          **178**

**Index**          **179**

# Preface

Again and again Jim and I have found that even highly intelligent people do all the wrong things with their dogs and end up with a canine delinquent on their hands! Behavioural counselling has always played a big part in my veterinary practice so that pups can become acceptable members of human families. Jim has gone on to train many of my puppy patients and has also unscrambled the behavioural problems of those patients who came to me too late.

I've always hated scientific jargon and have nodded through many a learned paper, reading the same line over and over again without taking anything in. Too often I have heard people complaining about their vets (and doctors) that they didn't have enough time to explain clearly what was the matter – or that they wouldn't or couldn't take the time to explain; or if they did take the time, you couldn't understand them, anyway!

So Jim and I decided it was high time that a clear and easy-to-read book was written by both dog trainer and vet – the first of its kind. We also decided it should be written without boring graphs and charts and in a light-hearted vein to demystify the wonderful world of communicating with dogs. Our aim of course has always been to ensure that dogs fit into their human pack without trauma to themselves or their well-meaning owners. Full of real-life anecdotes drawn from our experiences and coupled with a complete health guide, *Your Dog* offers an enjoyable and useful resource for all dog owners.

PART I

# Choosing Your Dog

# So You Think You Want a Dog?

## FITTING IN: DOGS AND THEIR OWNERS

### Families and children

'Mum, please can we have a dog?'

How many times has a mother heard this heartfelt appeal and put off the fateful moment with the frustrating answer, 'We'll see, dear' or 'Maybe one day'. It is, of course, a perfectly understandable reaction from any mother who dreads the extra load of chores that dog ownership seems to promise.

Bringing up a pup correctly to fit in as a happy, well-behaved and well-adjusted member of your family can be easy when you know how. It does require some time and effort, however, and if you cannot honestly spare the time, the result can be disastrous. A bored, neglected pup will quickly become destructive and your garden will probably look like an archaeological dig.

An important factor to consider is how a dog will interact with children. Should you happen to have a young child who is highly restless and energetic, then this could be overstimulating for a pup and you may well find yourself stuck with a permanently hyperactive dog. Most hyperactive dogs are made and not born as such for this very reason.

A young child can unwittingly make a dog's life hell. On the other hand, there are some dogs who absolutely adore children and only really come alive in their presence, tolerating all sorts of indignities such as kids swinging on their ears. Sadly, however, there are still hundreds of

3

dogs who wind up in pounds because they were 'bought for the kiddies', treated as a toy and then discarded when the 'fluffy pup' stage wore off and they started knocking the small children over in play.

Children must be disciplined to respect their pets. Even so, you can never be quite sure what's going on behind your back. Only when in her twenties did my daughter confess to me: 'Mum, remember when Twitchett had kittens and you showed me how to pick them up the right way and told me not to disturb them unless I asked? Well, I went straight back and picked them all up by their tails!' So be warned and keep a close eye on your children around their pets.

The real problem with children and dogs is that modern society has cut off most children from nature. Children today believe that watching a ladybird crawling on a leaf is strictly for the birds and they usually prefer computers to aquariums and pinball machines to picnics. All sorts of regulations, such as those banning dogs from school grounds, further segregate children from the natural (and canine) world, so it is not surprising that children often grow up scared of dogs and out of tune with their natural environment.

Apart from teaching the value of caring and responsibility, having a dog fulfils many childhood needs. Latchkey children coming home from school to empty houses have some of the scariness and loneliness taken away by the uninhibited welcome of a dog. Being accompanied by a dog on a leash makes it far safer for children who are sent out on errands. With the frantic lifestyles adopted by so many people today, parents often do not make enough time to listen and talk to their children, and a dog can act as an emotional safety valve.

Dogs make great listeners. I blanch, however, every time I hear someone say, 'My dog understands every word I say!' No, he doesn't. Don't kid yourself. Dogs appear to understand, and that is what is important to a child. Of course dogs can learn to associate the sounds of words with particular situations, but that is very different to actually understanding the meanings of words. Dogs pick up all the everyday words that they depend upon, such as 'dinner', 'lead' and 'walk', and a dog can thus acquire an impressive vocabulary.

The benefits of owning a family dog can be great but not if you cannot take the time for careful selection of your pup and for family co-operation in rearing him. Without this time and care, a dog will grow to become an aggravating liability instead of a well-adjusted member of your family.

## Couples

It is not only families with children who want a dog to complete the family circle. Couples often get a puppy as replacement for a child and much love and emotional commitment is invested in this new family member. However, there can be a break-up of the relationship, which results in a custody battle between the partners for the dog.

Such was the case with a gay couple I know who owned an Old English sheepdog. Ironically the dog had bonded closely to the partner who was not particularly fond of dogs. Consequently, the dog went to the other partner who had taken all responsibility for him. The poor animal, deprived of its object of affection, was not happy and, when left alone, indulged in behaviour indicative of stress: destroying things and howling. It took a lot of therapy to sort out the problem. The resulting mood swings of the owner also caused inconsistency in the handling of the dog, which upset the animal even further.

Occasionally a dog will take a dislike to someone who absolutely dotes on dogs. This is a risk you take if you give a home to a fully grown adult dog. John, a friend of mine, had lost his dog in a car accident and bought an adult dog to fill the emotional gap. He rang me up one day, quite distressed: 'I can't believe this! I have had dogs all my life and I get on well with them but this dog hates me. He's scared stiff of me. I've tried everything to get him to come around.' The dog appeared to get on well with John's partner but it was meant to be John's dog after all. Finally the vendor agreed to take the dog back. It was a sad case of the wrong personal chemistry – a doggie variation on the human situation where she loves him but he loves someone else!

## The elderly

A pet is sometimes the only lifeline elderly people have. Many of their peer group may have died and as a result they have few friends left. They may also suffer from severe, ongoing health problems. A sense of isolation may be further complicated by failing skills and feelings of not being needed, which reduce or threaten to destroy self-esteem.

A pet can fulfil some of these vital needs, sometimes in unexpected ways. One pensioner told me that her grandchildren visited her much more often now that she had a dog. For a person who is severely handicapped, a cat or a budgie would probably make a more suitable pet although arthritis sufferers often achieve increased mobility if they have to exercise their dog.

The choice of dog for an elderly person is very important. Too often an elderly person is 'pack-leadered', that is to say dominated, by her or his dog. And it does not even have to be a large dog.

Mrs Graham had an Australian silkie that had been spoilt rotten from puppyhood. 'That used to be my favourite chair,' said Mrs Graham, looking fondly at Spark who was sitting in it, 'but he goes for me if I try to take him off. And as for getting a nasty splintery bone away from him, I haven't got a hope. He sleeps on my bed now and scrapes at the door and barks his head off if I don't let him into the bedroom.' She said it all with enormous pride and love for her dog. 'What

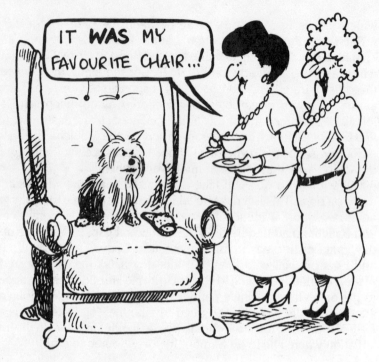

does it matter,' I thought, 'she is perfectly happy in her enslavement!'

With a larger dog in the same situation, however, it could be a more dangerous proposition. A cultured and gentle elderly European man came to see me with a 6-week-old bull terrier pup, a super dog full of character and with a good temperament. Even so, alarm bells started ringing in my head.

'I hate to say this but I honestly think that a bull terrier could be a bit much for you later on. He'll be a very strong dog both mentally and physically. Would you consider taking him back to the breeder? It would not be cruel to return him now as you have only had the pup a day and it has not bonded with you yet.'

There was no way he would consider it. The trouble did not start until Conker was about 5 years old. He had always had his own way simply because he had done nothing that was unacceptable to his owner so there had never been cause for a confrontation. He was, like all his breed, a stoic about needles and easy to handle in the surgery. Then one night he got a bone stuck across the roof of his mouth, right in the middle of a gripping TV drama.

He was no trouble when given an intravenous tranquiliser but after I yanked out the bone, which he regarded as a terrible affront, Conker leapt at me quick as a flash, missing the artery in my wrist by a mere dog's whisker. I warned his owners never to trust him again, but not long after this incident Conker bit someone who tried to pat him in the park. If authority and leadership had been established when Conker was still a pup, none of this would have happened, but the gentle temperament of his elderly owner was such that he could not give his dog the disciplined upbringing he so desperately needed.

### Young singles

Young singles often acquire a dog through either accident or impulse. A stray dog will wander into a shared household and, as often happens, no one takes direct responsibility for it so that even feeding is a hit-and-miss affair. Essential vaccinations, worming, registration and the necessary details of collar and lead all go by the board. Young singles in group accommodation also move on or go overseas, often leaving a dog that may have bonded with them strongly. These situations are difficult to avoid.

Although they may not make the ideal dog owners, at least young people, to their credit, are usually caring enough to see that a hungry, stray dog does not end up in the pound. It is to be hoped that local vets will be kind enough to give the same discounts to students and unemployed as they now do for elderly pensioners.

The young single who lives alone, often in a flat, should think twice before owning a dog. If you have a full-time job, the dog will be alone all day and this is very tough on an animal that is by nature a member of a pack. Unless a dog is raised in an exceptional manner, it is likely to suffer from separation anxiety, resulting in such problems as unacceptable urinary and defecation patterns, uncontrollable barking and destructive behaviour.

There are ways around this problem, such as the arrangements made for a Yorkshire terrier who became very special in the eyes of his mistress. On an early morning walk with her dog, this owner found she was being followed by a man. As her stride increased so did his, until finally she broke into a run and threw herself into the garage doorway of her block of flats. As the man went to grab her, the terrier flew at him and seized the ankles of the assailant's trousers with his jaws, upsetting the man's balance, and then barking furiously until the caretaker of the flats arrived to the rescue.

This diminutive canine hero, all 2.5 kilograms of him, was looked after during the day by an elderly pensioner. This was a fairly good arrangement as the pensioner's loneliness was alleviated without the responsibility and expense that is entailed in owning a dog while the dog had daytime companionship. In theory, however, it is not an ideal solution, as a dog who has its time divided between two people sometimes has a bit of an identity crisis deciding who its owner, or pack leader, really is! Ideally you should get your dog conditioned to being alone when you are out of the house. Always take it for a walk before you go to work in the morning to take the edge off its energy—and put an edge on yours!

## WHY OWN A DOG?
## ALL THE WRONG REASONS

The young, the elderly and families usually have a dog because they like dogs. The reason is as simple as that and, with the right guidance in upbringing, the result is nearly always a happy one.

Unfortunately, however, there are some people who acquire a dog for the wrong reasons. It can be sheer impulse, as in the case of the girl who one day saw an Afghan hound dashing across a park looking like a flying floccati rug. She went out the very next day and bought an Afghan without bothering to research the breed, or to consider her own circumstances. You do not leave a breed of dog, who is first cousin to the greyhound, locked up in a flat all day! The shift worker trying to get some sleep in the flat below thought it was Pharlap's ghost pounding around over his head.

Then there are the dogs that are bought for security. I was called to see a German shepherd because the owners 'could not get near him'. This highly intelligent dog had spent most of his life tied to a rotary clothes hoist instead of being reared as an exceptional breed of dog with special needs. The owners would have been better off with a burglar alarm.

There are also the status-symbol dogs, purchased because they are a rare and therefore impressive breed or they match the decor. It would be kinder for all concerned if this type of owner bought a pet rock! Some dogs are bought simply because they are very large and spectacular. I recall once seeing what seemed to be a driverless Mercedes Benz cruising down the street with an enormous Great Dane in the passenger seat. Out of the car climbed a small man who was obviously terrified of his dog, thus the dog had become pack leader and impossible to handle.

## THE DOG OWNER IN THE
## MODERN WORLD: PROS AND CONS

Being a suburban dog-owner today means having to put up with a lot of flak from 'pet haters'.

They are often people who are overemotional about health hazards without being well informed about the facts. Restrictions placed on dogs worldwide by new and harsher laws have given a lot of ammunition to this anti-dog faction; such people use it at every opportunity.

A woman was walking her dog up a none-too-tidy back lane when she was abused by an irate resident while her silkie was making a comfort stop by his back gate. 'How would you like me to come and do that outside your back gate?' he roared.

I have also been attacked for the same reason. A man hurled abuse and a handful of stones at my dog in mid-crap while I was actually standing beside her with a plastic bag at the ready to clean up. His aggressive attitude made me want to throw the contents of the bag at him!

The English-speaking communities are a lot more uptight in their approach to a dog's need to relieve itself than are the Europeans or Asians. In Paris, for example, there are mechanised turdettes (council cleaner-driven buggies that hoover up dog crap) and even doggy latrines on some street corners. In Amsterdam special bins are provided. Sweden has built blocks of flats with exercise yards on the roof, supplied with proper drainage systems to wash away excreta. And who but a Dane would win an award for designing a 'Pooper Scooper'. Singapore's exquisite orchid-filled botanical gardens allow leashed dogs. Labour is so cheap and it gives someone a job to clean up after your dog.

Everywhere you go nowadays there are 'No Dogs Allowed' notices and threats of penalties and fines. The fine for dog owners is as high as $1000 in one public venue in Sydney, Australia. The notion of your dog sharing your picnic with you in a park or the romantic idea of a run along a deserted beach with your dog rounding up the waves has become an impossible dream, although in Western Australia Cottesloe Beach has an area for unleashed dogs.

To be a modern dog-owner you must be responsible for cleaning up after your dog. Many places now carry on-the-spot fines for failure to comply with hygiene regulations, sometimes with sad results. In New York, fouling not howling was the number one dog problem of the city. In 1979 the Environmental Protection Department reported that 113 636 kilograms of dog excreta and 455 000 litres of urine were deposited on the public grounds and streets of New York that year. When the 'clean up after your dog' law came into being, the ASPCA (American Society for the Prevention of Cruelty to Animals) reported a 25 per cent increase in the number of surrendered dogs but even a maximum fine of $50 for dog owners did not make a picnic in Central Park a fragrant or inviting experience!

When walking your dog, you will have to acquire a thick skin to ignore public abuse so your outing will not be spoilt. There are, however, many positive aspects to walking your dog. You would not think for a moment of approaching a total stranger and asking what their favourite dinner was, but you would hardly be thought eccentric for saying to another dog owner, 'My, your dog does look very well. What do you feed him?'

There is a large and happy fraternity of dog owners who have an instant rapport; the very fact of sharing the experience of dog ownership makes an excellent gambit for conversation. That sure beats sitting in silence on a train journey without uttering a word to your fellow passengers!

I hope you still want to become a dog owner! If it is for the right reasons, you will not regret it.

# 2

# Pitfalls of Purchasing a Pup and How to Prevent Them

## 'MY-OTHER-DOG' SYNDROME

A prospective dog-owner who has had a much-loved dog before can suffer from 'my-other-dog' syndrome. In these cases, owners go to great lengths to expound the virtues of their previous pooch, which possessed an 'unblemished' record in all aspects of canine behaviour. We humans often seem to remember only the good points of dearly departed friends – canine, feline or otherwise. While this may be an admirable trait in some ways, please spare a thought for a new pup who is expected to live up to the exalted reputation of its predecessor. Enjoy your new pup for what it is, because every dog is different and every dog has its day.

## A HEALTHY PUP: THE SIGNS

If you have never owned a dog, it is very easy not to know what a pup in good health looks like. Some dog owners have never even taken in the normal details of their dog's anatomy. One panic-stricken owner turned up at my surgery, convinced that her dog had a bone tumour growing on top of its head. The 'tumour' was just a very prominent occipital crest – common in some dogs – where the two sides of the skull join together. Because the dog was a particularly hairy beast, the owner had simply failed to notice it before.

Here are some indications of a healthy pup. Whether crossbred or pedigree, pups should be fresh and alert when involved in their litter play. Between these playtimes, they should crash out in a relaxed heap to sleep. Their skin should look loose and elastic as if a few sizes too big, as this means there is a healthy layer of fat deposited in the skin layer. There should be no sign of a mucky bottom, denoting bowel infection or worms, and the eyes should be clear with no discharge. Check ears and nose for discharge too. The pup should not have bowed legs nor should the legs be 'cow-hocked' at the back, that is to say, with the legs turning outwards when it walks. Shivering or skin stretched tight on the bone are also warning signs of poor health in a pup.

# DECISIONS, DECISIONS . . .

## Male or female?

Some prospective owners have very definite ideas about whether they want a male or female pup. Others don't care one way or the other because they are ignorant of the specific problems relating to the sex of a dog. The reasons people give for their choices are varied and sometimes quite strange. While some prefer a dog of the opposite sex to themselves, others prefer one of the same sex. Too often these choices are related to the particular person's attitude to human gender and sexuality, rather than anything to do with dogs. But to make a sensible and informed choice, you should be aware of the real differences in male and female dog behaviour.

### Territory

Female dogs do not become as territorially oriented as do males and they do not mark out their territory. A female will not normally become aggressive with other dogs and will only search for a mate when she is in season. These factors make life with a female dog, particularly one who has been desexed, a lot easier than that with a male.

Male dogs are more egotistical than females and therefore show a more natural desire to mark out their territory as they mature. As an adult male, they will normally defend this territory against other males. Dogs have a unique and very distinct body language. When two male dogs meet and dispute territory, although a fight may not develop, in almost every case one dog will display dominance signals and the other a submissive attitude to settle the issue.

While most territories are restricted to where the dog lives, a dog who has been allowed the freedom of the street will continue to extend his territory by marking, thus creating a greater area to defend and in turn causing more headaches for the owner. This extension of territory will also occur if a dog, who is walked by the owner around the same route every day, is allowed to create scent posts along the way. This is how two male dogs of equal dominance, belonging to neighbours in the same street, can become arch enemies for life.

Such was the case with Toby, a Weimaraner who normally never fought, and James, a large, black, short-legged shaggy crossbreed. Crossing the street was the only way the owners could get past each others' houses. James and his owners eventually moved to another district. One day the owner of Toby, the Weimaraner, came to visit James's family. She deliberately parked her car well up the road, with Toby locked inside the car. James was not to be fooled (or foiled) this easily however and on the visitor's departure he dashed out, wild with rage, and chased her car while Toby rocked the car from side to side in his passion to tear apart his mortal enemy. Due to his blindly ferocious lunge into the road, poor James was run over by another car. Fortunately, he survived. It was clear that one suburb was not big enough for these two dogs.

This situation can be avoided. When walking to the park with a young male dog, keep him leashed and do not allow him to mark territory until you get there. This precaution somewhat decreases the strong territorial sense that the dog has for its own street.

## Sex

Undesexed male dogs will be interested in sex for 52 weeks of the year. Many misguided owners believe that if their dogs have some sex life it will cure them of an interest in sex and all the associated behavioural problems. Wrong! In the dog world, the rule is 'what he has not had, he will not miss'. Should you arrange a partner for him, you will be introducing him to a world of new and wonderful delights and he will be forever scaling fences in search of more female 'talent'. Thus you will have created a whole new set of problems for yourself!

Many male dogs embarrass their owners by being perpetual 'flashers' – and always at the wrong moment. One lady told me she had decided to have her dog desexed. 'Why?' I asked. 'He's not a fighter.'

'I'm just fed up with him flashing,' she replied. 'And not only that. It's smelly and messy. Why just the other day I was driving along in the car and off he went, sitting right next to me. I knew I'd cop the lot so I grabbed a bunch of paper handkerchiefs to cover the offending part. Then I saw this fascinated busload of tourists looking in at me while we waited at the traffic lights. Must have thought we were a weird mob! No, I can't tolerate it any longer. He'll have to be desexed,' she said firmly.

Can't say I blame her!

## Large or small?
### Small

Most small dogs have a large dog inside them, trying to get out. They can have indomitable courage, strong wills and plenty of arrogance. They are also more active and more capable of hunting, munching up large bones and taking long walks than you would ever suspect, judging from appearances. On the other hand, they are cheaper to feed than bigger dogs. You don't have to climb over them when you're trying to do the cooking, like I have to with my Weimaraner. And you can smuggle them into all sorts of places where dogs are normally not allowed.

Once I saw a tiny round basket on a window ledge in an exclusive restaurant. A smart couple sat eating at the window table, which was level with the ledge. I wondered where the man had been 'dragged up' when he picked up some pâté on his fingers. His lack of manners was soon explained when his wife furtively raised the basket lid and a tiny mouth popped up and took the delicious morsel!

### Large

Big dogs make their presence more obviously felt by their sheer size. A wag of a Labrador's tail can sweep ornaments off a coffee table, but once they are mature – which can take up to two years – Labradors are very quiet around the house. Breeds like the Irish wolfhound, which dropped to alarmingly low numbers during the Second World War due to food shortages, have made quite a comeback in the United Kingdom. They stroll around the block with great dignity and seem content spending a lot of time lying about looking decorative. In contrast, the small terrier is always bounding with energy and rearing to go.

## COSTS AND CARE

Some pedigrees, especially if rare, are extremely expensive. Costs of pedigree dogs will often vary according to public demand. Phone around several breeders to check prices and ask how much it is to buy a pedigree as a pet without papers. This is if you do not want your pet to be a show dog as it may have some small fault, in the coat marking for example, which does not detract from the dog's health but would tell against it in the show ring. You could not breed from such a dog and sell the pups with registration papers.

The price for pups without papers should be much lower than for those with papers. Sometimes breeders will sell cheaper if the owner guarantees that he will not breed from the dog but will have it desexed. Or you may come to an agreement with the breeder to let the bitch have one litter with the choice of pup to the breeder. Make it clear just what deal you want and make sure you get it in writing.

**Expensive hairdos**

Caring for some breeds can cost precious time and money. Devoted Afghan hound owners sometimes splurge on Mason Pearson hairbrushes and many dogs' coats need conditioners after shampooing. Larger dogs, of course, take more shampoo. Remember that dog bath-products cost much more than human preparations because of the chemicals used. Trying to economise by using human shampoos will often result in a dog scratching himself to pieces because the Ph balance is not right.

Time must be set aside for caring for a long coat. There is no sadder sight than an Old English sheepdog covered with knots; I saw one Maltese terrier whose foot hair was so badly knotted that its feet resembled four tennis balls.

# 'WHERE DID YOU GET THAT DOG?': SOURCES

Here are a few handy hints and precautions according to where you purchase or acquire your pup.

### The friend's bitch who was 'got at'

You will have some idea how these pups are going to turn out because you do know the dam (or mother) and even the identity of the sire (or father), fleetingly glimpsed as he was chased off into the sunset by the bitch's owner. This will give you clues as to how the pups will look, what their temperament will be like and if they came from healthy parentage. But bear in mind the famous conversation between George Bernard Shaw and a beautiful American actress when she proposed marriage to him with the suggestion that they would have enviable offspring given her exceptional beauty and Shaw's exceptional intelligence. Shaw declined, pointing out that their children could well end up with her brains and his looks! Genetics can play funny tricks.

### Pounds

Why does a dog end up in a pound? It may have strong roaming instincts and like to go 'walkabout'. Having no identity disc due to the negligence of its owner, the dog then gets picked up by the dog-catcher. On the other hand, it may be a 'mother's darling' who never moves a paw without the mistress but who slips out one day when a tradesperson accidentally leaves the gate open. It also may be surrendered to the pound because of some behavioural defect but, in many cases, questionable behaviour has been prompted by a stressful environment and owner neglect. Often such dogs, who are badly behaved, will adjust readily to a kind new owner who offers affection and a secure environment.

A client rang me one day. He had hitherto owned only cats. 'We have just got the most wonderful German shepherd from the pound. He has a super temperament and is quiet and house-trained. We'd like you to check him over.' It sounded too good to be true. I could not fault him. But why was he in a pound?

We soon found out. The next day the new dog-owners went out to their part-time jobs. On returning, they found the garden looked like an archaeological dig and the back door was in shreds – an obvious case of separation anxiety. After time and patience, we trained the dog out of this condition and, as he became more secure, he did indeed become the 'perfect' dog.

Jim Fraser has trained countless crossbreeds from pounds and many have become model pets. On the debit side, some dogs have had behavioural problems that have required extensive modification through training before they became well adjusted. These behavioural problems are not, however, limited to dogs purchased from pounds and can be found even in expensive purebred dogs and in dogs purchased from private sources.

If you do not want a dog for show or breeding then the pound is a good place to start your search. For a start, you will be saving a dog's life. Also, the price is usually very reasonable. Many pounds have vets who examine, vaccinate and, when the animal is old enough, desex your dog – all included in the purchase fee. Not only are crossbreeds available but pedigree dogs as well.

On the down side, puppies especially can undergo extreme stress in a pound, often producing a breakdown of the dog's immune system with resultant diarrhoea from parasites, viruses or simply due to the stress itself. Many pounds do have a health guarantee and often the pups are vaccinated but sometimes this does not prevent a puppy from getting sick after purchase as it can take some ten days for a pup's immunity to develop its full strength after vaccination. This time-lag might fail to beat the challenge of virulent infections, always present in pounds.

This is exactly what happened to the Hammond family's pup. 'It was perfectly healthy when we got it two days ago. Six weeks old, chubby and bouncy. Now it's skin and bone with terrible diarrhoea, utterly depressed and won't eat,' said a worried Mrs Hammond. The puppy had to be maintained on a drip for several days and it was a long hard pull to get it well again. The pound authorities were prepared to treat the pup under their written guarantee but the Hammonds lived too far away from the pound to make this a practical proposition.

Other people purchasing from a pound actually want to hand back a pup when it gets sick as if it were a pair of trousers to be returned because the zip got stuck! Such people should not be dog owners. The average person, once she or he has purchased a pup, feels a deep commitment to it as a creature with feelings and the ability to suffer; as a result, a firm emotional bond is almost instantly established. Pounds can be the suppliers of some of the most endearing dogs imaginable. There is also the immense satisfaction of knowing that you saved your dog's life. But keep your wits about you. A guarantee should cover enough days to allow for an incubating disease to become apparent.

**Pet shops**

Pet shops can be very dubious sources for both pedigree and crossbred pups. The premises may appear very clean but the rapid turnover of young, disease-susceptible livestock can cause disease to be endemic. It would be unwise to purchase from a store that does not give a health guarantee like the type discussed above.

There are many good pet shops whose reputations suffer only because of the bad name of a handful of others. Take note if the premises are clean. It is a good sign if the shop owner has the pups behind glass where they cannot be constantly handled and scared by the public, and where stressful noise can be cut down. This shows that the owner has some knowledge of the fragility of a pup's health and takes a caring, sensitive attitude to his or her animals.

Staff in a pet shop should know something of the background of the pups but it remains a problem that you cannot view at least one of the parents. Nevertheless, *do* check the pup's age, which ideally should be 6–7 weeks at the time of purchase. Pups that have not been socialised with people by the age of 10 weeks may never accept humans without showing some sign of fear. So beware of that little puppy huddling in the corner for it may turn out to be a 'fear' biter. Pups undergo a fear imprint between 8 and 10 weeks, which means that indiscriminate handling at this time could be such a bad experience that it could stay with them for life. It is best therefore to avoid pups over the 8–10-week age bracket if they display obvious signs of neurosis. Pet stores can establish good reputations by taking whole litters of pups from breeders to sell on a long-term, ongoing basis.

**Market places**

These are highly dubious sources from which to purchase a pup. A large percentage of pups purchased from markets become sick, often fatally. The market environment is the 'perfect' set-up for lowering a pup's resistance to disease: just taken from its mother, jammed into a cage that may be infected with viruses, hyped up by the busy market atmosphere and handled by too many people without adequate rest or proper food.

# CROSSBREEDS AND PEDIGREE DOGS

**The much-maligned mongrel: the crossbreed**
It was one of those late-night emergency calls when I ducked out of the shabby entrance of a rooming house in the inner city. I had just been to see an old pensioner's dog that had been run into by a boy on a skateboard and now the poor animal could not stand up. As I headed for my car, past the pub at closing time, a man lurched out onto the pavement in a drunken haze, snarling 'You bloody mongrel!' at someone.

Safely inside my car with the reassuring presence of my large dog, I pondered on the drunk's use of the word 'mongrel'. 'Mongrel', 'cur', 'bitch' are favourite terms of abuse. 'How ironic,' I thought, 'that we malign animals who live by a code of behaviour that rarely makes them as fatally aggressive as their so-called "best friends", us humans. And what a great shame it would be if there was no such creature as a "mongrel" or, to use the correct term, "crossbreed".'

Despite their undeserved reputation, crossbreeds are a very necessary part of the canine world. Because there has been no close breeding with relatives, crossbreeds are less likely to have inherited physical and mental defects. What's more, your crossbred dog will be a totally exclusive model. There will be no other quite like it in the world. Think how people misguidedly pay for some rare and overvalued commodity when you can get a unique crossbreed for nothing.

Admittedly, some crossbreeds look like that children's game where you can flip over the cardboard tops, middles and bottoms of different animals to get all sorts of crazy mixed-up creatures. Sometimes it seems that God was having a bad day when he assembled the parts! The results can certainly be outrageous, like the offspring I once saw of a long-haired dachshund and a female shaggy-haired, long-legged bitch. Their owners did not imagine such a mating was possible but dog's aren't stupid and love always finds a way – after all, there was a flight of steps in the back garden!

One problem of purchasing a crossbreed is that it takes a bit of guesswork to know how it will turn out, but if you study our pup selection test (page 25) you will at least have some idea of its temperament.

**Pedigree dogs: a short history**
In the days when men were men and women, bashed on the head with a brontosaurus bone and tugged by the hair, were not glad of it, a dog was a dog. If they could talk, they would tell us they were glad of it because since those cave-dweller days, people have stretched the dog into strange shapes called breeds.

What did this original dog look like? As much as anyone can intelligently infer, this ancestral dog had a neat, compact body. It had straight legs, which were longer at the back than the front for speed and propulsion to catch its dinner on the hoof. It had a broad head to accommodate enough grey matter to be intelligent, longish jaws to seize prey, eyes that looked directly to the front to spot the slightest movement in the undergrowth and pricked ears to tell the direction of any sounds. These ears also allowed plenty of airflow to discourage the growth of germs and the accumulation of any waxy discharges. The tail was long to act as a rudder when swimming and to help balance when on the run. If the climate was cold, the coat would be heavier and the tail bushy, curled around the dog's body when asleep, to conserve heat.

So how did different breeds of dogs come about? Humans and dogs first got together at least ten thousand years ago. We know this from dog bones found around the sites of kitchen middens in Scandinavia dated to this time. Dogs evidently made useful 'garbage disposers' by eating rotting refuse. It would be sentimental not to admit that dogs were eaten too but primitive people soon found out that dogs could be invaluable to their survival. Being fleeter of foot than humans, dogs could find and chase game and then hold it at bay until the cave dwellers caught up to club their 'dinner' to death. The dogs no doubt got handouts and when fire was discovered, a circle of dogs probably would gather, round the camp fire, attracted by the tantalising smell of sizzling meat. Even today, dogs usually get a drooly, glassy-eyed look when they smell a roast cooking. The cave dwellers' dogs also acted as guards against large predators. From a hunter's tool to a fireside dinner guest, the dog slowly worked its way into the inner circle of human company. No doubt, one day a puppy was given to a child as a plaything and an even closer relationship was built between human and beast.

During these primitive times there would have been groups of dogs that were better at the chase while others were better at sniffing out the quarry or made more trustworthy guard dogs. In this way, some natural selection took place. But then humans began deliberately breeding dogs for their particular strengths and skills. All ancient civilisations had their huge hunting dogs; the hunt was the sport of kings and for a long time was thought to be a more fitting pastime for young noblemen than poetry or the other arts. For this royal 'pursuit', the fast movers of the greyhound type were developed.

The huge, powerful mastiff-type dogs were bred to be used in bear-baiting and warfare. The Romans took them from England and used them for protecting their military supplies and the rearguard of their armies. They did sentry duty and, in the frontline, wore armour and could bring down a man on horseback. Henry VIII sent 400 of these warrior dogs to help King Charles V of Spain in his war against the French.

And so, by human design and needs, breeds of dogs came into being.

Some were a ghastly mistake. Take the Pekingese – its short, bowed legs and squashed face with popping eyes were an error of nature, a genetic mutation that the ancient Chinese seized upon and developed through intensive inbreeding. The Pekingese has now become one of the most popular breeds in the world today.

Where did it all go wrong? What probably seemed like a good idea at the time has produced many freaks of nature. Humans went overboard, creating new breeds of dogs by selective breeding. Breed characteristics became overexaggerated resulting in actual discomfort for the dog. So we ended up with the British bulldog whose squashed face makes breathing an effort; the Hungarian puli, lugging around a coat of Rastafarian dreadlocks; spaniels with ears dangling in their dinner; Pekes with popping eyes that get pinned on rose-prickles and basset hounds with cabriole legs that would look more sensible on a Queen Anne chair.

The too-close shuffling of genes to fix, that is to say breed true, a so-called desirable type often resulted in dogs being born with inherited physical and mental defects. The list is as long as your arm. The most common hereditary condition is hip dysplasia, where the ball and socket joint in the hip does not fit properly, resulting in crippling arthritis. Other horrible genetic problems include retinal atrophy causing progressive night blindness; lids that roll inwards to irritate the eye; lids that roll outwards so that a dog looks like it had a bad night on the tiles; haemophilia; tiny pieces of genetically misplaced skin tissue growing on the surface of the eye; a whole host of bone malformations; and epilepsy, just to mention a few.

As a dog owner, be aware that these problems exist and that there are caring and conscientious breeders who have worked hard to stamp out such defects and to modify some of the more exaggerated physical characteristics. In terms of health, the most trouble-free breeds of pedigree dogs and crossbreeds are those that most closely resemble the primitive dog, such as the dogs of Southeast Asia and the Australian dingo.

## SELECTING A PEDIGREE DOG

All breeders suffer from 'kennel blindness'. There is no breed quite like theirs – perfect in looks and temperament and never puts a paw wrong! Of course there are plenty of individual dogs around like this but certainly not all members of a particular breed. In some countries a certain breed may have a bad reputation while in others there will be a different line of the same dog that enjoys a good reputation. Much may depend on where a breed originated and whether there are bans on imports in a particular country, resulting in heavy breeding programmes from the limited stock available.

When some breeds become fashionable, this can create an unnaturally high demand for those breeds. At one time the corgis of British royal family fame took on like wildfire so that the ankles of not only the royal household enjoyed nips from these little Welsh heelers of cattle. Television stars like Lassie created the fashion and consequent high demand for collies. Unsuspecting collie owners, not realising what they were in for with the dog's long coat to look after, tossed many a poor animal out on the street. The pounds ended up with more than their fair share of beautiful collies. Once a breed becomes popular, many breeders get on the bandwagon and churn out 'assembly-line' pups that are bound to be poor physical and mental specimens. Because the bitches have not been allowed a rest between whelpings, the pups are often scrawny with poor bones.

Breeders' descriptions of dogs can read like real-estate advertisements – with similar traps for the unwary. In the same way that 'harbour glimpses' means you can see the ocean if someone dangles you out the attic window by your ankles, so too does 'aloof with strangers' or 'shows great affection for the family' probably mean that the dog bites! When I read the following description of a Weimaraner, 'He is at his

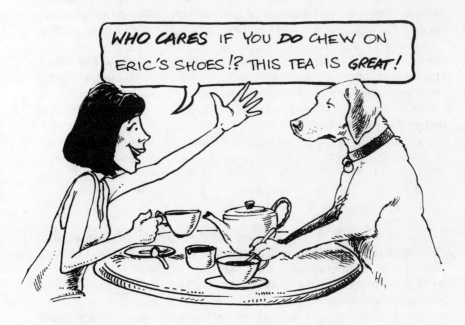

*'He is at his best when allowed to share family life as a responsible member . . .'*

best when he is allowed to share family life as a responsible member with a job of work to do', I wondered if he'd put the kettle on and make me a cup of tea!

Volumes have been written listing all the dogs in the world. Breeds are categorised differently in each country. The British, American and European kennel clubs differ as to how they group the breeds and how many groupings they list. And there are many breeds we have not heard of in the English-speaking world, such as the smalandsstovare, the griffon a poli laineux or the wetterhund. So, if you have a wonderful 'Heinz-fifty-seven-variety' bitser and someone asks you what breed it is, you can look them straight in the eye and say, 'It's an applestrudelhund!'

With this vast selection from which to choose, it makes good sense for the prospective owner and all the family to peruse as many books as possible from the library. The origin of the breed and its historical background can be easily researched but unfortunately there is little said about the pitfalls of particular breeds. My next chapter goes some way towards filling this gap.

## BUYING A PEDIGREE PUP

First of all, never be in a hurry. Don't be like the Kramers. They decided they must get a pup in two days because it was young Jamie's birthday. A mad rush around a handful of breeders and they ended up with a dog of the opposite sex to what they wanted and with a nervous temperament as well. The dog wound up always trying to bite Jamie out of fear because Jamie's main aim in life was to be Rambo and Superman rolled into one; he was constantly on the move, leaping off things and very effectively imitating the sound of a machine-gun. Even a normal, well-adjusted dog would have been hard pressed not to have a nervous breakdown!

So please don't make the Kramers' mistake. For a start, ring your local kennel control body and get the name of the secretary of the breed club and its address. Contact them for information on the breed you have chosen and what litters are available. Breed clubs also often have literature available and they hold open days when you can get detailed information.

The next step is to try to visit the kennels before the litter of pups is ready to leave its mother. This way you can watch the litter and see which dog's temperament is most suited to your needs.

When I suggested this to the Morrisons, Mrs Morrison said, 'But it's half a day's drive to the place! We haven't the time!'

'It's very little time,' I warned her, 'when you consider that you will be spending the next ten to fifteen years or so with this dog. If you make a mistake now and get the wrong dog for your needs, you will eventually resent the animal, which will react adversely to your feelings of resentment and the whole experience of happy dog-ownership will go sour. Believe me, it's time well spent!'

Happily, the Morrisons took my advice.

## VISITING THE BREEDER

Even if you have a registered breeder's name from your local kennel control, you may still be in for a bit of a culture shock when you visit the kennels.

The premises are ramshackle, the breeder greets you with fingernails in which you could plant potatoes, his clothes are dirty and muddy, the house smells appalling and there are heaps of old, rotting newspapers piled against the walls. 'I'm not buying from here!' you think indignantly, wondering how to make a quick getaway. In fact, you might have struck one of the best breeders imaginable and, remember, you are buying a *dog* and not a *property*! Some breeders could not care less about their personal surroundings or appearance but they care greatly about their dogs.

Note one thing however: are the pups raised on a back verandah or in a room inside the house? A litter raised in an inside room may be stimulated by household smells and be used to voiding inside the house. A dog from such a litter will be conditioned to this routine and may prove an absolute nightmare to house-train! On the other hand, a litter raised outside will naturally relieve itself outside so that the house-training will probably be a breeze. There is nothing worse to spoil your relationship and your carpets than a dog dirty in the house.

Some breeders have so-called 'championship stock', which you might have seen in the show ring. So, you go to the kennels and are shown a dog from this line. But what you do not know is that this 'champion' got high points at country shows where it was the only one of its breed being exhibited! One buyer ended up paying the earth for a Newfoundland that looked as if a steamroller had run over it.

Some owners will look you up and down with a steely eye. Mr Garside was a business tycoon, used to giving commands with no answering back. His entrepreneurial nature got a pounding when a little lady bustled out of the kennels and said, 'Now, if you're not going to walk this dog when it's grown up at least one and a half hours a day, you're not having it!' He did not have it – which was probably just as well. You must expect a grilling about your suitability as a dog owner and take it in good faith even if the enthusiastic dog breeder has never attended charm school and learnt good public relations.

Beware of the puppy factories. I went with a friend to pick up a dog that was in need of a home. She was an old breeding collie no longer needed for this purpose. This fact in itself spoke volumes about the attitude of the breeder. The place was spotless, the house festooned with silver cups and red, blue and green ribbons. The kennels were filled with ferocious-looking shepherd dogs who obviously had not been socialised.

While the breeder went to fetch the collie, a family was waiting to buy a pup to become a guard dog. I struck up a conversation with them, which made me realise that they did not have a clue about dogs and did not in fact like them. As I suggested in a low voice that maybe they would be better off with a burglar alarm, out walked the breeder with the collie. The wretched dog was flat-footed, cow-hocked and its poor old bones had degenerated from having too many puppies. She looked so sad. I said to my friend, 'You realise you are getting a dog who is a physical wreck and probably about 8 years old!'

She took the dog. I would have done the same thing in her place. It was love at first sight and the dog enjoyed a few happy years with her new owner. But not I think the poor puppy that the breeder sold to the family. Off they went without a word of instruction from the breeder about its welfare or their ability to fulfil that dog's needs. The poor child screamed as she walked past the harmless old collie. I left there with a sinking feeling in my stomach. The breeder had got his money and that obviously was all he cared about.

Another beautiful German shepherd, ruined in this way, was bought as a guard dog by a family who were told by the breeder to leave it locked up in the garage and not to fondle it in any way. Lack of socialisation and training made that dog totally unapproachable. There was even a limit to what an experienced trainer like Jim could do for it.

## SELECTING FROM THE LITTER

Once you have decided that this breeder, warts and all, is fine for you and the pups seem healthy and happy, you need to select *one*, even if you want them all.

Watch the pups at play. The litter bully is often the first one to prance over to the edge of the pen to greet you. Lots of buyers are caught this way. 'Why, look! He chose me!' Yes, I've already heard that statement literally dozens of times. The buyer is sold the dominant pup of the litter, which ends up pack-leadering their little Henry and later picking him up by the pants!

Then there is the one in the corner. It has been left out of the normal litter play and is isolated and already harbouring behaviour problems that will affect its adult life. This dog is a submissive, stressful type of pup that will need careful and thoughtful handling to build confidence and character or with the wrong kind of handling it will be a 'fear' biter.

You wouldn't be human if you weren't attracted to a pup visually. Certain markings can be appealing as well as the size and colour of the pup, but unless you investigate further the dog can end up like a frock or a suit you adore that does nothing for you once you actually wear it. Here are a few rules-of-thumb for selecting a puppy for suitable temperament and character.

First, watch the litter without them seeing you. Then watch with them seeing you. Then you can subject the one you fancy to the following simple puppy test. You will need an area just outside the pen and away from the rest of the litter. As a courtesy, explain to the breeder why you want to do this.

# THE PUPPY TEST

### Social attraction
Put the pup on the ground and move a little away from it. Then clap your hands. Does the pup come towards you, tail up and happy, or does it tentatively creep over to you with its tail held low? This test indicates how sociable and confident the pup is. If it takes no notice at all, it is likely that it has a strong independent streak that could become quite a problem later on.

### Following
Walk away from the pup slowly and steadily in one direction. If the pup follows, what does it do? If it bounces around in front of you playfully this means that it is confident. If it grabs your trouser leg, swings on your skirt or makes to chew your feet, it will probably turn out to be a 'bossy boots' and will want to pack-leader the whole family. But it is just as likely to make a great dog as a security guard or in obedience trial work, given the right owner.

Some pups trot after you tentatively as if scared to be left behind. These pups are lacking in confidence and need to be near a leader. Some pups thumb their nose at you and act as if you were not there at all. This indicates independence of a kind that you do not want in a dog as it may be virtually untrainable.

### Elevation dominance
Cradle the pup in your hands, which are placed on either side of its body, and gently elevate it to about half a metre above the ground. The pup is now entirely under your control. Does it wiggle and squirm, fighting back strongly to escape your enfolding hands to get back to

terra firma, or does it just plop there quite passively? This will tell you if the pup is going to accept the owner as boss.

## Social dominance

Everybody thinks that dogs just love to be stroked on the head. This is in fact not true. To a dog this action is a very dominant gesture. Stroke the pup gently but firmly from the top of the head to down the neck. Dominant pups do not accept this treatment and jump up, getting out from under the hand and often biting at it. Others just stalk off, showing total independence. The more submissive ones accept the stroking.

## Restraint

Roll the pup onto the ground gently and hold it there with a hand on its chest for about 30 seconds. If the pup hates to be dominated, it will thrash around, biting at your hands and trying to get up. Others just flop there.

All these tests are only *indications* of the tendencies of a pup's personality but they are reliable enough to avoid getting a totally unsuitable pup for someone such as a child or an elderly person. A pup's behaviour will show modifications from its personality type according to its reaction to its new environment. In this way, a stable home environment can calm and give confidence to an overanxious pup to some extent while a stressful environment can make the most placid pup neurotic. Remember, your pup may be a genetic marvel but, with the wrong approach, you can fail to mould it into a happy and disciplined dog and waste its potential to be the perfect pet.

# 3

# A Handy Guide to the Breeds

## DON'T JUDGE A POOCH BY ITS COVER: PEDIGREE DOGS

A dog that develops behaviour problems is very often a pedigree breed that has been bought on impulse without properly researching the suitable breed for its particular owner. Don't we all know what trouble falling for good looks can lead us into? Dig deep below the attractive packaging and you often find defects of character you'd never dreamt of, or else traits that are just different from what you'd expected. Then you are disappointed and the chances of building a close relationship are shattered. The result – rejection, leading to anti-social behaviour. This applies to men and women as well as people and their dogs.

In this chapter I give broad outlines of the types of dogs available and brief descriptions of the different breeds, so you won't fall into the trap of buying the wrong dog for you, with all the heartache that follows. All figures given for standard heights for each breed mean height at the shoulder. Heights given are the maximum for dogs; bitches are slightly smaller. Sometimes breed standards only show heights or weights and not both, which can be misleading when you think of say the basset hound who is only up to 38 cm high but a big dog who happens to have short legs! The groups described are according to Australian Breeds Standards. Each part of the world classifies dogs differently, which is very confusing. For example, a dog might be classified as a 'worker' in one country and as a 'utility' in another.

Dogs mentioned as being 'spitz' originated in the Arctic Circle. All have thick woolly undercoats, straight harsh top-coats, bushy curly tails, prick ears and a somewhat wolflike appearance.

# THE TOYS

Most toy dogs are absolute little charmers. They are past masters at the art of manipulation, usually managing to blackmail their owners to get what they want. The royal courts of England and Europe were inundated with little dogs, the small spaniels being especially popular. The famous seventeenth-century diarist Samuel Pepys commented after a visit to the Council Chamber of Charles II, 'All I observed was the silliness of the King playing with his dog all the while and not minding the business'. Dogs had some practical value too. Another literary work of the time speaks of 'The smaller ladyes poppes [puppies] that bear away the fleas and divers small fowles'. So, it seems that in Olde England toy dogs were used as flea traps.

Most toy dogs have overcrowded mouths that can lead to tooth problems; the Australian silky terrier, however, is less prone to this condition. Many but not all toy breeds are strong willed so, if spoilt, can learn to use their teeth on their owners.

**Affenpinscher**   This breed has a gorgeous little face like a monkey, and is referred to by the French as a moustached devil. It is comical and affectionate and may originally have been a member of the 'Pinscher-Schnauzer Klub' in Germany. Never underestimate the toy dogs; they will walk you off your feet if that is what you like. This breed makes a good watchdog.
*Height*   Up to 28 cm.
*Weight*   Up to 4 kg.
*Colour*   Black is preferable but grey shadings are permissible.

**Australian Silky Terrier**   A diminutive cross between an Australian terrier and a Yorkshire terrier, the silky can match any dog for courage. It makes a great little guard dog. Two silkies were known to fell a burglar by grabbing at his trouser legs and running in different directions; even tight jeans did not deter them!
   This dog often lives to a great age. As the name implies, the silky's coat is long and silky.
*Height*   About 23 cm.
*Weight*   Up to 4.5 kg.
*Colour*   Blue and tan or grey-blue and tan.

**Bichon Frise**  Look out for the bichon frise in the paintings of the Spanish artist Goya. Descended from the ancient water spaniel, these dogs were adored by the French and Spanish aristocracy and were introduced to the Canary Islands by Spanish seamen. You must learn to look after the corkscrew-curled, white coat; this will take time as the dog should ideally look like an animated powder puff. It has a delightful disposition.
*Height*  Up to 28 cm.
*Colour*  White.

**Cavalier King Charles Spaniel; King Charles Spaniel**  The King Charles spaniel probably originated in Japan but became famous in the court of King Charles II. In those days it actually looked more like the present-day Cavalier King Charles spaniel, which is heavier and has a longer nose than the King Charles. These dogs were known as 'comforters' at court; indeed it seems His Highness took more comfort from them than he did from his two-legged friends, allowing the bitches to whelp and suckle in court, making it, according to Samuel Pepys, 'a nasty stinking place'. That dogs were indeed safer and more loyal friends than people is suggested from the fact that a King Charles spaniel remained huddled in the skirts of Mary, Queen of Scots after her execution. It would not leave her even at the point of death.

The King Charles spaniel is known in America as the English toy spaniel. In recent times the Cavalier has suddenly become very popular and in high demand so there are many Cavaliers that are not up to standard physically or mentally. Nevertheless both the Cavalier King Charles and the King Charles spaniels are delightful breeds and make ideal family pets. Just look for strong bone and good temperament.

Benny, a Cavalier King Charles spaniel and one of my favourite patients, was being trained by Jim Fraser who, much to the owner's surprise, described him as an arrogant dog. Benny did emit very strong personality vibes. This instigated a totally unwarranted attack from a savage large crossbreed while one of Jim's experienced dog walkers was exercising Benny. The walker saved Benny's life when he was seized by the throat. Benny came out of the attack unscathed and undaunted. Only the dog walker and vet suffered from shock.
*Weight*  Cavalier King Charles: up to 8 kg; King Charles: up to 6.3 kg.
*Colour*  Black and tan: raven black with bright tan markings; ruby: whole coloured rich red; Blenheim: rich chestnut markings on pearly white ground; tri-colour: black and white with tan markings.

**Chihuahua**  This is the smallest dog in the world and resembles nothing so much as a bonsai fawn. It is a brilliant guard dog, highly intelligent, easy to transport and cheap to feed so that it makes an excellent pet for the elderly. Despite its size, a chihuahua can walk for miles, attack any size dog and pack-leader its owner to an alarming degree. Doting lovesick owners are not in the least put off by being bitten for not toeing the line for their dog.

Originating in the state of Chihuahua in Mexico and named after that state, these dogs graced the cooking pots of the American Indians and were involved with religious, possibly sacrificial, rituals of the Aztecs. In more recent, happier times one was presented, concealed in a bunch of flowers, to the opera singer Madame Patti by the President of Mexico, and the famous conductor Xavier Cugat conducted with one tucked under his arm.

Their habit of shivering makes it appear that the chihuahua's owner is a cruel monster but, in fact, they do easily feel the cold and a dog coat is a good idea in winter. (There is also a long-haired variety of chihuahua.) In spite of their ability to enjoy long walks, they don't mind hitching a lift, like one of my patients who goes around in a shopping stroller. Handling him in the surgery for minor procedures such as cutting his nails necessitates the wearing of large motorbike gloves. Startled clients look at me as though I am tackling a tiger in there!

Because they are the smallest and most popular toy dog in the world, the high demand and intensive breeding mean that there are many poor specimens around so look out for good strong bones.

*Weight*　Show specimens should not be more than 1.5 kg.
*Colour*　Any colour or mixture of colours (no, not hot pink!).

**Chinese Crested Dog**　This is another rare but recognised breed that is almost completely hairless except for the feet, tail and head, where the crest may be flowing with locks. The skin needs regular oiling to prevent cracking and should not be exposed to too much sun. It is a hardy and lively dog and the skin normally feels hot to touch. It loves its owner and has a nice temperament.

*Height*　Up to 33 cm.
*Weight*　Up to 5.5 kg.
*Colour*　Any colour or combination of colours.

**English Toy Terrier**　This breed is known in the United States as the Manchester terrier (toy). In England and Australia, however, the Manchester terrier is a separate and larger breed from which the toy version descended, probably with some Italian greyhound blood introduced to miniaturise it. Although a part of English heritage, it is sad that English toy terriers have declined in popularity and there are not many very good specimens of this tiny smooth-coated dog around. It is a one-person dog.

*Height*   Up to 30 cm.
*Weight*   Up to 3.6 kg.
*Colour*   Black and tan.

**Griffon Bruxellois**   Cab drivers in crime-ravaged cities should take note that this dog started its working life in the front seat of Brussels taxis where its cocky personality came in handy for the drivers' protection. Descended from the ragtag and bobtail dogs of the Brussels streets with probably the German affenpinscher, this unusual breed has a squashed, bewhiskered, monkey-face and is one of the few toy dogs without a patrician background. This has not stopped it from becoming popular in high-society circles today.

It is tough, happy, intelligent and long-lived. There is a smooth-coated variety called the brabancon, which arose from a griffon crossed with a pug.
*Weight*   Up to 4.9 kg.
*Colour*   Clear red, black, or black and rich tan without white markings.

**Italian Greyhound**   This breed is total elegance in miniature, easily trained and very clean about the house. Although it therefore makes a good town pet, it needs plenty of off-leash exercise. It also feels the cold easily and needs a warm, knitted coat for winter. Never raise your voice to one as they are extremely sensitive dogs.
*Weight*   No more than 4.5 kg.
*Colour*   Black, blue, cream, fawn, red, white or any of these colours broken with white.

**Japanese Chin**   Looking rather like the Pekingese, this dog also has its origins in China, where the Emperor presented a pair as a gift to the Emperor of Japan about a thousand years ago. Queen Victoria, who was dog mad and did much to popularise the toy breeds, made these dogs fashionable so that British sailors, who have not changed much over the years, used to bring these exotic dogs home to sell. They are tough little dogs, sometimes known as Japanese spaniels.
*Weight*   Up to 3.2 kg.
*Colour*   Black and white or red and white.

**Lowchen**   This is a tough little dog with obscure origins. Its coat is cut to resemble that of a lion. This dog was thought to be favoured by the Duchess of Alba as a dog of similar appearance is shown with her in a portrait by Goya.
*Height*   Up to 33 cm.
*Weight*   Up to 3.2 kg.
*Colour*   Any colour or combination of colours.

**Maltese** Although probably not originally from Malta, this dog's history of being isolated on the island meant that it was genetically undiluted and thus bred pure for centuries. Highly prized in the most opulent and cultured period of Maltese history, these dogs finally became popular worldwide. Much was written about them in ancient Greek texts, including a short history of the breed by Aristotle. Nobles even erected monuments to their departed Maltese dogs.

This breed has a happy disposition and its white, cascading coat needs a daily bristle-brushing.
*Height*　Not over 25.5 cm.
*Colour*　Pure white.

**Mexican Hairless Dog**　This is an ancient, almost extinct breed, probably originating in Northeast Asia and brought to Mexico by nomadic Indian tribes. The Aztecs thought of them as a gift from the gods as they could warm the body of a sick person with their skin – dog hot-water bottles in effect. The body temperature of this breed is much higher than that of other dogs and they must be kept in a warm atmosphere. They are not a recognised breed in Australia.
*Weight*　About 13.6–16 kg.

**Miniature Pinscher**　Fondly known as 'min pin', this dog has absolutely no connection with the Dobermann but is a much older breed, descended from the German smooth-haired pinscher. It is essentially terrier in nature and a very sporty character, well muscled, fearless and can make an excellent guard dog. It has a gait like a hackney horse. It is also the most well constructed of the toy dogs.
*Height*　Up to 30 cm.
*Colour*　Black, blue or chocolate.

**Papillon**　The breed is so called because the erect fringed ears, with the blaze in the middle of the forehead, makes it look like a butterfly. This toy spaniel originated in either Spain or the East and became popular at European courts; it is often seen in this setting in the paintings of Rubens and Van Dyke. It ranked among pets of the French and the famous. Madame de Pompadour owned these dogs as did Marie Antoinette (I often wonder how her dogs fared when she was sent to the guillotine!).

Papillons tend to be devoted to their owners. Their delicate appearance belies the fact that they live to a grand old age and like plenty of exercise. A pet name for these baroque-looking dogs, other than 'butterfly dog', is 'squirrel spaniel' as the long, feathery tail curls right over the back, squirrel-fashion.
*Height*　Up to 28 cm.
*Colour*　White with patches of any colour except liver.

**Pekingese**   This ancient Chinese breed has a history probably better documented than that of any other breed. The Chinese were on to a good thing when the peke first made its appearance because the short, bowed legs and squashed face are really products of a genetic mutation (one of Nature's errors); they turned out however to be a blessing in disguise because the peke became one of the most popular and delightful breeds imaginable, living to a grand old age. In the imperial Chinese court they were looked after by the emperor's eunuchs who vied with each other to breed the best ones for their master; this competitive breeding was no doubt made more so by the fact that the eunuchs were not into that sort of thing themselves!

Pekes were also traditionally known as 'sleeve dogs' as some emperors carried them in the sleeves of their royal robes; often the colour of the dog matched the garment, for example a cream-coloured peke with a yellow robe.

The first pekes came to England by means of British troops, who had ransacked the Summer Palace in Peking in 1899 and stolen these dogs despite fierce resistance. Among those dogs presented to Queen Victoria, one peke was aptly named 'Looty'.

Pekes are quite fearless; their other title as 'lion dogs' was not earned for nothing. The long coat needs daily care and the eyes are particularly vulnerable to damage because they bulge.

*Weight*   Up to 5 kg.
*Colour*   Coat and markings, all colours.

**Pomeranian**   This is the tiniest of the spitz dogs and takes its name from Pomerania, a region of central Europe. Being a spitz dog, it probably originated in the Arctic Circle. It almost usurped the peke for popularity in its time. Like all the toy dogs, there is a much larger dog trying to get out and it tends to be a bit yappy. The thick undercoat and long overcoat, typical of the spitz dog, make it look like a ball of fluff.

*Weight*   Up to 2 kg.
*Colour*   All colours.

**Pug**   This is an unusual toy dog in that it definitely resembles a mastiff in miniature, with the same solid musculature. The face is wrinkled and squashed so that it can sometimes have similar breathing problems to the bulldog. This is not the toy for you if you like your pet in the bedroom with you, unless you're happy to wear earplugs when it snores!

The pug undoubtedly came from the East and arrived in Britain with William and Mary of Orange when they ascended the throne. After a decline in the pug's popularity over the years, Queen Victoria revived interest in the breed, which became a darling among artists. Hogarth owned one little creature who was the subject of a number of sculptures by fellow artists and was eventually immortalised in ceramic from the Meisen factories. They are great with children.

*Weight*   Up to 8.1 kg. (Watch it! They are gluttons.)

*Colour*   Silver, apricot, fawn or black.

**Yorkshire Terrier**   Yorkshire people are famous for breeding all sorts of animals from canaries to dozens of breeds of dogs; the background of this terrier does not even pretend to be nobly ancient. It is probably derived from the Skye and the Cairn terriers; history varies according to the particular text. The long silky coat is steel blue and tan. In spite of its size, it is a tough little dog.

*Weight*   Up to 3.1 kg.

*Colour*   Steel blue and tan.

# THE TERRIERS

In feudal England the mastiff was one of the giant breeds owned by the wealthy lords. In order to stop them poaching deer, the peasants were not allowed to own a large dog; they were permitted only those dogs that would fit through a wire loop of a certain dimension. If they needed a large guard dog, at the perimeter of a great forest, for example, law required that its claws be removed with a chisel.

Then in came the developers and reformers and chopped England into a patchwork quilt of fields during the agricultural revolution. Crops were grown on these tiny plots and were promptly eaten by weasels, stoats and rabbits. It was then that a small spunky dog came into its own.

'Another sorte there is which hunteth the fox and the badger and grey onely whom we call terriers: they creep into the ground and by that means make afrayde, nyppe and bite the fox and the badger in such sorte that they eyther teare them in pieces with their teeth, beying in the bosome of the earth, or else hayle and pull them perforce out of theyr lurking angles, darke dungeons and close caves.' This description, taken from a treatise written in 1576 on 'Englishe Dogges' (by Dr Paine, a 'Doctor of Physiche in the Universite of Cambridge'), aptly describes the terrier.

Gradually each country sported its own type and the terrier became the pride of the working classes – whose sport on Sundays was killing the vermin around the factories, in an age when England had become dependent on coal and steel. Before this profusion of local variants, of course, there tended to be only a few types of terrier but what they all possessed was the ability to dig into the ground after their quarry with enormous persistence, to seize it with strong jaws, and to kill it with a powerful neck shake. Terriers have sharp eyesight to spot creatures moving slightly in the undergrowth and they also possess the ability to turn quickly. They all have a formidable set of teeth, which usually never need scaling all their lives. Deprived of a busy outdoor life, they tend to mutilate themselves by scratching and, like any bored dog, will overreact to the cavortings of a single flea.

A dog-sitter looking after a Sealyham terrier in a small New York apartment had enormous difficulty persuading him to take a walk. The poor dog was so fat his square back could have served as a coffee table. He looked more like a toy dog on wheels, and he probably wished he had some. This is a sad fate for a dog with such an active background.

Most terriers weigh between about 7 and 15 kg. The largest of the terriers is the Airedale at 25 kg and the smallest is the Australian at 5 kg.

**Airedale Terrier**   This is the biggest of the terriers, probably originating from the old black and tan and the otter hound. They are fearless guard dogs and some of the finest I saw in the North of England belonged to a breeder in her eighties. Here, they were lounging on their own leather suite (what was left of it) in their very own sitting room.
*Height*   Up to 61 cm.
*Weight*   Up to 25 kg.
*Colour*   Body-saddle black or grizzle; all other parts, tan.

**American Staffordshire Terrier**   Although derived from the English bulldog and Old English smooth terrier, this breed is not to be confused with the English Staffordshire bull terrier, which is much lighter, although they were once one and the same. They were known as pit dogs when first in America, since they were derived from dog-fighting stock; nor is this breed to be confused with the unrecognised pit bull terriers, which are American Stafford, bull terrier and mastiff crosses bred for fighting and which should be banned, but are in Australia 'underground'. These dogs can be extremely dangerous to people, whereas the American Staffordshire is normally great with people, but fights with other dogs.
*Height*   Up to 48 cm.
*Colour*   Any colour – solid, parti-colour (partly one colour, partly another or other colours) or patched.

**Australian Terrier**   This breed is hugely popular as a pet in Australia. It was hard for breeders to fix a type as it came from quite a cocktail of British terriers. They are supposed to be derived from a Yorkshire terrier smuggled in in a lady's muff. They are good with people but, as is characteristic of all terriers, they will give a cat a good run for its money!

*Height*  About 25 cm.
*Weight*  About 6.5 kg.
*Colour*  Blue, steel-blue or dark grey-blue, with rich tan on face, ears, under body, lower legs and feet and around the vent.

**Bedlington Terrier**  The Bedlington is a very pretty terrier, looking rather like a lamb with a tucked-up waist that probably came from the introduction of whippet blood some years ago to give the dog more speed. The Bedlington's head curves from forehead to nose in an unbroken line and its rather mincing appearance denies the fact that, like all the terriers, it can hold its own in a scrap.

*Height*  About 41 cm.
*Weight*  Up to 10.4 kg.
*Colour*  Blue, liver or sandy with or without tan.

**Border Terrier**  This is one of the most entrancing of the terriers – small enough to go to ground after a fox and long-legged enough to follow the horses. It is a very quiet house dog, although it can run rings around you on a country walk. It is not aggressive with other dogs, needs plenty of space for exercise and is not nearly as popular as it deserves to be.

*Weight*  Up to 7.1 kg.
*Colour*  Red, wheaten, grizzle and tan or blue and tan.

**Bull Terrier**  Until bull baiting was banned in 1835, this terrier was bred as a bull baiter and dog fighter by crossing the bulldog with the terrier to give it more speed. The bull terrier has an undeserved reputation, as most are affectionate with people and devoted to children, but some are unreliable, possibly because they have been incorrectly handled by their owners. If they bite, they hold and are reluctant to let go. No better pet if you buy the right strain.

*Height*  Up to 48 cm.
*Colour*  White; for coloured varieties, may be with white or brindle.

**Bull Terrier (Miniature)**  These are derived from smaller bull terriers.
*Height*  Up to 35.5 cm.
*Weight*  Up to 9 kg.
*Colour*  As for bull terriers.

**Cairn Terrier**  This was a working dog developed on the Isle of Skye. It was used to flush out otters and foxes from among rocks, hence

its 'rock' name. Although a very lively character to have in the city, this terrier makes an excellent house dog.
*Height*   Up to 31 cm.
*Weight*   Up to 7.5 kg.
*Colour*   Cream, wheaten, red, grey or nearly black.

**Dandie Dinmont Terrier**   Low to the ground with its soft top-knot and soulful eyes, this dog's appearance belies its tough terrier disposition. The breed was named by Sir Walter Scott, who based his novel *Guy Mannering* on the real-life character James Davidson of Harwich. Called Dandie Dinmont in Scott's book, this man was the proud owner of a number of these terriers.
*Height*   Up to 28 cm.
*Weight*   Up to 11 kg.
*Colour*   Various shadings of pepper or mustard.

**Fox Terriers (Smooth and Wire)**   Of all the various breeds derived from the more general sort of terrier, the smooth and wire fox terriers are the most popular. They have been bred with a rather narrow head and resemble a child's toy dog without the wheels. Goitre, glaucoma and dislocated lenses can be inherited problems in a few.
*Height*   Up to 39 cm.
*Weight*   Up to 8.25 kg.
*Colour*   White predominates with black, black and tan or tan markings.

**Glen of Imaal Terrier**   An Irish working terrier.
*Height*   Up to 36 cm.
*Weight*   Up to 15.9 kg.
*Colour*   Blue, brindle or wheaten.

**Irish Terrier**   This breed is larger than the fox terrier, and of course it's a redhead with plenty of fire.
*Height*   Ideal is 48 cm.
*Colour*   Red, red wheaten or yellowish red.

**Jack Russell Terrier**   This dog was only recently recognised as a breed and has become enormously popular.
   The famous hunting parson, the Reverend Jack Russell, bred these dogs in Devon, where he died well over 100 years ago. Terriers were selected small enough to go in the huntsman's saddle bag, from where he would take them out and set them to ground in pursuit of a fox. I remember seeing these small dogs years ago with the head huntsman of the Devon and Somerset Foxhounds, a pack reputed to

be stopped only by a gate or a pub! These dogs have all the spunk, energy and personality of the terrier group.

*Height* The larger version – the Parson Jack Russell terrier – is nearly 10 cm taller than the Jack Russell terrier, which is 25–30 cm.
*Weight* 1 kg per 5 cm of height.
*Colour* White must predominate with black, tan or brown markings.

**Kerry Blue** Another type of terrier from Ireland, this dog is sporty, a good guard and likes scrapping.
*Height* Up to 48 cm.
*Weight* Up to 16.8 kg.
*Colour* Shades of blue, with or without black points.

**Lakeland Terrier** This terrier comes from the English Lakeland district, which used to be a popular hunting area. It looks a little like a small Airedale.
*Height* Up to 37 cm.
*Weight* Up to 9.5 kg.
*Colour* Black and tan, blue and tan, red wheaten, red grizzle, blue or black.

**Manchester Terrier** A black and tan terrier by the name of Billy was reputed to have killed 100 rats in eight minutes in the rat pit, the working man's sport in old England's mining towns. From this type of dog came a more fined-down version – the Manchester terrier. These excellent ratters certainly dispatched the rats in a faster, more humane way than did the slow process of poisoning. Times were often hard for the working person in industrial England so the family terriers from towns would often be used to catch a rabbit for the stew-pot. They make a good house dog.
*Height* Up to 41 cm.
*Colour* Jet black and rich mahogany tan.

**Norfolk and Norwich Terriers** These were the good old low-to-the-ground type of terriers, who excelled at digging out their quarry. Cambridge University students, on their days off, would go vermin hunting with these dogs and be able to keep them as pets in their lodgings. How ideas of leisure have changed! They are good-tempered house pets.
*Height* Up to 26 cm.
*Colour* Shades of red, wheaten, black and tan or grizzle.

**Sealyham Terrier** The smart, white Sealyham will hunt in a pack. Fanciers of the breed in England thought it was being spoilt by the

easy life of the show bench, so they formed the Sealyham Terrier Badger Digging Association to keep this dog's working ability up to scratch! The Sealyham is quite obstinate and can be a fighter.
*Height*    Up to 30 cm.
*Weight*    Up to 9 kg.
*Colour*    Mostly white, sometimes with other markings.

**Skye Terrier**    This breed is the glamour pants of the terriers with a long, hard top coat and hair that hangs from the edges of its ears like a fringe. The Skye terrier has a steel-trap jaw, which is most effective if it decides to fight. This dog was made famous by the story of Greyfriars' 'Bobby', the dog who stayed by his master's grave for 14 years, leaving only to visit the cafe, where he used to go with his master, to be given a bun every day. A statue of this loyal dog has been erected on its grave.
*Height*    Up to 26 cm.
*Colour*    Black, grey, fawn or cream – all with black points.

**Soft-coated Wheaten Terrier**    This is another of those Irish terriers without the formal trim, as its coat falls in waves or casual curls. It is an all-rounder who can kill vermin, be a good guard and gun dog and is fine in the house.
*Height*    Up to 49 cm.
*Weight*    Up to 20.5 kg.
*Colour*    Like ripening wheat.

**Staffordshire Bull Terrier**    Because of unfortunate mishaps with bull terriers and the deserved reputation of pit bulls, people are misguidedly scared of Staffordshire bull terriers.

A senior citizen at a bus stop looked horrified when one of my patients, Jose, who was sitting outside a shop, spotted me and hurled herself at me to cover me with kisses. The pensioner thought my end had come!

Great family dogs – I've never met one who was bad with people, but some, especially the male, do love a good dog fight. They are derived from the bulldog and probably the Old English black and tan terrier.
*Height*    Up to 40.5 cm.
*Weight*    Up to 17 kg.
*Colour*    Red, fawn, white, black or blue, or any one of these colours with white.

**Welsh Terrier**    This terrier looks a little like a small Airedale, is a fiery redhead and a potential fighter.

*Height*   Up to 39 cm.
*Weight*   Up to 9.5 kg.
*Colour*   Black and tan or black grizzle.                    •

**West Highland White and Scottish Terriers**   These terriers are
sadly more familiar on the label of a famous brand of Scotch whisky
than they are in real life. The West Highland White is more outgoing
than its reserved cousin.
*Height*   Up to 28 cm.
*Weight*   Up to 10.4 kg.
*Colour*   Scottish terrier: black, wheaten or brindle of any shade.

# THE GUN DOGS

It is a bizarre fact that this group, bred for the country gentry, are among
the most popular town pets. The reasons for this are their striking good
looks and the adoration with which they regard their owners.
Historically, gun dogs have had a very close relationship with their
aristocratic so-called sportsmen owners, usually ranking higher than the
wife in their affections and working closely with them in the field. Their
main aim in life is to please. It is therefore not surprising that this group
of dogs needs people!

I acquired my Weimaraner because he was not allowed in the house
of his owners in the country and he went 'walkabout', looking for company. He ended up choosing us. The owners eventually asked me to
take him as they were tired of collecting him from all over the district.
It was therefore with misgivings that I took this dog to a built-up city
area but it says something for his choice of new owners that, back in
the country with the door open, he does not want to go for a walk unless
we go with him!

People must play a big part in the lives of a city-slicker sporting dog,
otherwise it can turn to petty crime. Out of the frustration of sniffing
only suburban concrete, being restrained on the end of a lead, and often
being left lonely in a backyard, these dogs will become acutely miser-
able. The Labrador who already displays a too-broad waistline will
escape his 'prison' and upturn garbage cans, sublimating his misery
by stuffing himself with rotting food!

The more energetic sporting dogs may become overactive and sometimes destructive. Many will sit and chew themselves out of boredom,
resulting in *lick granulomas* – sores that can become cancerous.

The transformation of the sporting dog when it gets taken to the
country is miraculous to behold, so if you opt for one in the city, get
it to an interesting park with bushes, trees and space every day. Also

make sure you have it in the house with you. People almost make up for everything natural these dogs are deprived of, living in the city. Owning such a dog is a heavy commitment indeed!

## The Pointers

Yes, they do point! 'Hey dad, look! There's a duck over there' is what they are saying in effect when they freeze and point their head on outstretched neck with one foot raised in the direction of the game. This breed came about in the mid-seventeenth century before the sport of shooting birds in flight became popular. The pointer located game, such as hare, which was then chased by the faster greyhound, who did not possess a good enough nose to sniff out the prey. The foxhound, the greyhound and possibly a bit of bloodhound all contributed to the making of the pointer, probably around the same time in several European countries, especially in Spain, as well as in its traditional home of England. By the end of the seventeenth century, the pointer was being bred with more dash but less of the killing instincts of the greyhound and foxhound blood. They are great dogs in the house.

The pointer has the following characteristics.

*Height*   Up to 69 cm.

*Weight*   Up to 34 kg.

*Colour*   Black and white, lemon and white, liver and white, self (i.e. plain, all one colour) or tri-colours.

*Trainability*   Late maturers and can lack concentration as they are easily distracted.

**German Short-haired Pointer**   This type was bred from a German pointing dog that had its origins almost certainly in the Spanish pointer, to which English pointer blood was introduced. Great gun dogs and household pets, they retain a delightful youthfulness even in their dotage, as witness my old friend Jake, who is 14 and has survived having tick poisoning, heartworm, an ear amputation, an eye removed and a broken leg! He behaves like a puppy, perpetually cheerful and undaunted!

*Height*   Up to 64 cm.

*Weight*   Up to 32 kg.

*Colour*   Solid liver, liver and white spotted, liver and white ticked, liver and white spotted and ticked, or black and white.

*Trainability*   Very active dogs and late maturers, sometimes lacking in concentration, and easily distracted.

**German Wire-haired Pointer**  This pointer made a very handy and versatile hunting dog; it had to switch from pursuing duck to pheasant to hare to deer, all in a day's work.
*Height*  Up to 67 cm.
*Weight*  Up to 34 kg.
*Colour*  Liver and white, solid liver or black and white.

## The Retrievers

**Chesapeake Bay Retriever**  This is an American breed little known outside the United States – a tough working retriever with none of the glamorous looks of many American dogs. In 1807 a British ship was wrecked off the coast of Maryland and everyone aboard was rescued, including a black bitch and a red dog who both appeared to be Newfoundlands. The dogs were given to the man who sheltered the shipwrecked seamen. He found that both dogs had terrific retrieving ability. By outcrossing the dogs (that is to say, not breeding them together), the Chesapeake Bay breed was fixed in another 78 years. The breed is of course named after the site of the shipwreck.

This retriever is famous for its coat, which is short and dense, with a woolly undercoat; with one shake, the water showers off because of the oil. It is tough, steady and a good house dog.
*Height*  Up to 66 cm.
*Weight*  Up to 34 kg.
*Colour*  Of fading grass or wet sedge, which acts as camouflage, and in the summertime the coat goes the colour of the shedding coat of the buffalo.

**Curly-coated Retriever**  An ancient breed of water dog in Europe, covered in Shirley Temple curls, was the originator of this breed into which slipped some poodle blood. It is a very strong dog that can endure hours in freezing water; the little air pockets between the tight curls keep it warm.
*Height*  Up to 68.5 cm.
*Weight*  Up to 36.3 kg.
*Colour*  Black or liver.

**Flat-coated Retriever**  This breed was produced from the Labrador and the Newfoundland. It has a dense, flat coat.
*Height*  Up to 61 cm.
*Weight*  Up to 35 kg.
*Colour*  Mostly black, sometimes liver.

**Golden Retriever** Although now very popular, this is a comparatively recent breed, coming from a mixture of Newfoundland, spaniel and setter and originating from a mutation of a flat-coated retriever. It is docile and gentle, great with children, sensitive and easily trained.
*Height* Up to 61 cm.
*Weight* Up to 36.3 kg.
*Colour* Shades of gold or cream.

**Labrador Retriever** Of all the retrievers, the Labrador is the most popular and deservedly so, having made its mark as one of the best gun dogs, guide dogs for the blind, PAT (Pets as Therapy) dogs and household pets. When you have a Labrador puppy you won't believe a word of this because they are late maturers and, until then, can be destructive, and they love wandering. But hang in there. In two and a half years you will have a dog as described in the books!

Labradors have a superb temperament and are great attention seekers. They go about this in such a nice way that they always get what they want, which partly accounts for the high rate of obesity among Labradors.

In the early nineteenth century, fishermen visiting Newfoundland saw these smaller retrievers working well with wild fowl. The Earl of Malmesbury imported some dogs into England and from these the breed developed worldwide.

Many of the Labradors in establishments such as nursing homes are reject guide dogs. A reject army-tracker dog was my house guest for a year when his owners were overseas. We soon found out why he was rejected. His nose was remarkable and he would go off in hot pursuit of a scent but never come back! By the time the owners returned we all looked like Twiggy.
*Height* Up to 57 cm.
*Weight* Up to 34 kg.
*Colour* Black, lemon or yellow that ranges from light cream to red fox and there are a few chocolates.

**Nova Scotia Duck-tolling Retriever** You might suspect that the average duck would give a wide birth to a dog! Apparently not the Nova Scotia ducks who are lured through curiosity to within gun range when the hunter lies hidden and throws sticks for his dogs to play with on the beach! Then the toller is sent out to retrieve the dead or wounded duck. Intelligent and easy to train, these dogs must retain this playful trait. A double coat protects them from icy water.

*Height*   Up to 51 cm.
*Weight*   Up to 23 kg.
*Colour*   Various shades of red or orange.

## The Setters

The setter's origin was most probably from spaniels and Old Spanish pointers. The name came from the fact that when these dogs saw game they would sit, or set, while the owner got his or her act together.

**English Setter**   This setter's coat is longish and silky with a feathery appearance around legs and tail. A gentle disposition typifies the English tweedy country gent's dog.
*Height*   Up to 68 cm.
*Weight*   Up to 30 kg.
*Colour*   Black and white, lemon and white, liver and white or tri-colour and often flecked.

**Gordon Setter**   This breed is a very hard worker and not a bit flashy.
*Height*   Up to 66 cm.
*Weight*   Up to 29.5 kg.
*Colour*   Black and tan.

**Irish Setter**   As one might expect, this dog is a flaming redhead with temperament to match. It is reputed to be flighty but this rather maligns it because it is highly intelligent. A late maturer, it is very receptive to training but this must be in the hands of the right person as Irish setters tend to be cunning; and, if you succeed in training them well, cunning dogs can turn out to be the best of the lot.

The thing about setters, especially the Irish, is that they all work on a wind scent, mostly on open moorland. So beware, for when they catch an interesting whiff on the breeze they are off! It is this behaviour that gives them the reputation of having no road sense.

I remember a leggy lady being towed into the surgery on the end of an Irish setter one day. 'Can you give him something to calm him down?' she pleaded. Personally, I thought it was her who needed the tranquillisers.
*Colour*   Red chestnut; white on chest, throat, chin or toes, or small star on forehead or streak on nose.

**Irish Red and White Setter**   This setter has a base colour – pearl white with solid red patches; it may have some mottling or flecking.

## The Spaniels

The spaniels are an ancient group dating back to the fourteenth century when they were either land or water spaniels.

**American Cocker Spaniel** This dog is an eye-catcher with immensely long ears and cascades of hair that make it look as if it is wearing a grass skirt on each leg. In spite of this bizarre appearance, its sporting instincts are still very active, although I would not fancy cleaning one up after a muddy outing! Freddy, a patient, is one of the most enchanting dogs I have met, but he is a walking genetic disaster with his inherited ear and eye problems.
*Height* Up to 38.75 cm.
*Colour* Jet black, black and tan, brown and tan or parti-colour.

**Brittany Spaniel** Britain lays claim to being the originator of so many gun dogs when in fact they all came from Europe! Many European popular sporting dogs never got a foot in the United Kingdom. Thus it was with the Brittany spaniel, which has more the build of a setter than of the English spaniel; the latter has become shorter in the leg over the years. The Brittany is now one of the most important bird dogs in the United States.
   This French breed is an excellent all-rounder, will both retrieve and point to find game, and is friendly and intelligent.
*Height* Up to 52 cm.
*Weight* Up to 15 kg.
*Colour* Orange and white, maroon and white, black and white, tri-colour (black, white and tan) or marked with one or other of these colours.

**Clumber Spaniel, Field Spaniel** The short-legged clumpy clumber spaniel and the field spaniel leap from tussock to tussock in the field. Both breeds are larger than the cocker.
*Height* Field: up to 45.7 cm.
*Weight* Clumber: ideal, 36 kg; field: up to 25 kg.
*Colour* Clumber: plain white body with lemon markings, can be orange; field: black, liver or roan, or any one of these with tan markings.

**Cocker Spaniel, Springer Spaniel** The cocker spaniel came from the land spaniels and hunted woodcock. Other spaniels sprang the game, that is they sent it airborne so the falcons could get it; hence, they were called springer spaniels.
   Cockers are very good with children. They also have a look, with eyes that seem to melt, that can slay your heart. They love

communicating with other dogs, often in a noisy way and, although very easy to train, they do take offence easily so you must be particularly gentle with them. An occasional strain of cocker bites without warning.

The long ears can knot easily so they should be brushed daily and the insides checked for excess wax as they tend to pick up infections. Old spaniels get heavy wrinkled brows so that they can hardly see. Some spaniels get infections in the folds, or 'flews', on the sides of their mouths, which can smell very nasty.

*Height*   Cockers: up to 41 cm.
*Weight*   Cockers: about 14.5 kg; springers: up to 23 kg.
*Colour*   Cockers: various colours; springers: liver and white or black and white.

**Sussex Spaniel, Welsh Springer, Irish Water Spaniel**   Certain districts have their spaniels too, such as the Sussex spaniel and the Welsh springer. The Irish water spaniel is much bigger than other spaniel breeds and is covered with ringlets. The **American water spaniel** is similar to that of the Irish, but it is not a recognised breed in Australia.

*Height*   Sussex: up to 41 cm; Welsh springer: up to 48 cm; Irish water spaniel: up to 58 cm.
*Weight*   Sussex: 22.7 kg.
*Colour*   Sussex: rich golden liver; Welsh springer: rich red and white; Irish water spaniel: rich dark liver with purplish tint.

## Other Gun Dogs

**Hungarian Vizsla**   The vizsla was little known outside its native Hungary until many people fled the Russian occupation during the Second World War and took their dogs with them. It is a quiet, clean house dog, and a good all-rounder that is fast and clever.

*Height*   Up to 64 cm.
*Weight*   Up to 30 kg.
*Colour*   Russet gold.

**Italian Spinone**   Popular both as a gun dog, working well in woods and marshes, and on the show bench, this breed originated from a number of ancient French breeds – mostly hound and pointer types. The coat is harsh and shaggy, especially around the head, and I nearly made the faux pas of mistaking one for a ragtag and bobtail London bitser, which was sitting quietly in the waiting room of a Central London smart vet practice and belonged to the receptionist. They are

good natured and quiet, excellent with children, have a sweet expression and yet are good guard dogs.
*Height*   Up to 65 cm.
*Weight*   Up to 39 kg.
*Colour*   Mainly white, or white with orange or chestnut patches.

**Munsterlander (Large)**   Usually breeds are refined down to get smaller versions but in this case the breed was evolved from some of the larger Small Munsterlanders, having the build of a setter and the head of a spaniel. The multipurpose gun dogs are easily trained, affectionate and reliable, and well adapted to rough conditions.
*Height*   Up to 61 cm.
*Weight*   Up to 29.5 kg.
*Colour*   Always black and white with black head and patches or flecks.

**Weimaraner**   Known as the 'grey ghost' because they are all the same silver-grey mousey colour with amber or blue-grey eyes, the Weimaraner was bred in the court of Weimar, Germany, in the nineteenth century. The sameness of the breed is due to the fact that the German breeders rigidly culled litters and guarded the breed so jealously that no dogs were allowed outside Germany. The objective was to produce a dog that was a good all-rounder, unlike other gun dogs, which are each specialised in a certain field. An American with great persuasive powers managed to join the exclusive Weimaraner club and finally took two back to America.

This powerful hunter is definitely not a dog to be left in a yard as it can suffer from stress through isolation, a condition common in sporting dogs.
*Height*   Up to 69 cm.
*Colour*   Silver-grey, shades of mousey grey.

## THE HOUNDS

When you look at a page of pictures of the hound group, they make a very odd assortment: long legs, short legs, pointy jaws, chunky jaws, svelte or heavy, hairy or smooth. Although they all make great pets, generally not expressing any aggression towards people, they do in fact possess a strong killing instinct and each type works in the hunt in a different way.

The long-legged ones are fast and will sight, catch and kill their quarry; others, like beagles, hunt by scent alone and their heavier physique makes them stayers, able to track over huge distances. Some hounds give 'tongue', which means they make a heck of a racket until the hunter arrives to dispatch the prey. Then there are those with a low-slung chassis like the dachshund, who go to earth and find the prey until the hunter comes along and digs them both out. When Oscar Wilde described hunting as 'the unspeakable chasing the uneatable' he probably wasn't referring to the dogs! Generally speaking all hounds need plenty of exercise and may have a tendency to worry livestock.

**Afghan Hound** Reputed to be an aloof dog, some Afghan hounds have become nervy and withdrawn through no fault of their own. Their glitzy appearance – with the cascades of long silky hair on body and ears and with their oriental-looking eyes – has made them popular in the fashion world and jet set. Afghans are 'sight' hounds, which means they see, rather than scent, their prey.

Some stories say the princes of Afghanistan hunted leopards with these dogs. The females were let out of purdah to act as a decoy by jumping on the leopard's back while the male went for the quarry's throat. They also were used to hunt with the hawk, who would land on and agitate the prey, such as an antelope, so that the Afghan could catch up and hold it at bay until the hunter arrived.

Like all hounds, they have a mind of their own and are not that easy to train. One tends to see Afghan owners being dragged along by their Afghan hounds.

*Height* Up to 74 cm.

*Colour* All colours.

**Basenji** This African hound, with the worries of the world written on its wrinkled forehead and a tail like a Chelsea bun, was much prized by natives in the Congo. They hunted with basenjis in packs to drive game into a net. The basenji was also known as the *M'bwa m'kubwa M'bwa Mamwitu* or 'jumping-up-and-down' dog because it could leap up vertically in the long grass to spot game; it wore a wooden rattle to indicate its whereabouts. A remarkably clean, odourless dog, it washes itself like a cat. It does not bark but 'yodels'.

Independent and inscrutable, it is hard to train because it does not indicate by body language what it is thinking. This dog has the distinction of being one of the few dogs that has ever bitten me. Even so, they are nice with their own family, including the children.

*Height* Up to 43 cm.

*Weight* Up to 11 kg.

*Colour* Pure red or black, or black and tan.

**Basset Hound** The basset is a scent hound that was developed after the French Revolution for use by the poorer people, who hunted on foot, brandishing firearms. If you were to put legs of proportionate length on a basset, you would have an awful lot of dog. They were bred so low to the ground to get through rough undergrowth and, as a result, their ears dangle in their dinner.

They are, perhaps, not overendowed with brains but then, who needs them with such a charming personality! Avoid the model with cabriole legs pointing outwards in ballet number five position. They are not the easiest dogs to train either.

One client's basset would only come when she played the flute. He escaped from her car one day in the stock exchange area of Sydney. So out came the flute. I waited for a line of stockbrokers to come, as if summoned by the Pied Piper of Hamelin, after the returning basset!

Some bassets who come to the veterinary practice have to be seen to be believed. They collapse and go all floppy. Not believing in ever using forced restraint, I went through a whole packet of biscuits one day just to cut a basset's toenails. You get the best results training them with a light, jolly approach.

*Height*   Up to 38 cm.

*Colour*   Generally tri-colour (black, white and tan), or lemon and white.

**Beagle**   Because this is a small hound with a neat, attractive appearance and nice personality, people are sometimes deceived as to its true characteristics. It is a hound, after all, and a trot around the block twice a day is really not enough to keep it fit and content. Thus many beagles become obese.

I am reminded of the sad sight of three such unhappy dogs, kept in the backyard in an inner city suburb; they had awful fights with each other out of sheer frustration. Being a member of a pack, as of course all dogs were originally, these dogs need you as their re-placement 'pack'. It is lucky that they are clean and quiet around the house once they are mature and are then best kept inside as they tend to be very destructive in the garden. They are not easy to train: Jim describes them as four legs and a tail!

*Height*   Up to 40 cm.

*Colour*   Any hound colour but not liver; always has white tail-tip.

**Black and Tan Coon Hound**   This all-American hound developed from a number of European hound types. It is used to hunt, mostly at night, for possums and racoons; it moves fast in the dark, hunting by scent, and then traps its quarry up a tree, giving tongue until the human killers arrive. It is not a recognised breed in Australia.

**Bloodhound**   A most unfortunate name for one of the most huggable, sooky dogs imaginable. Its early reputation as bloodthirsty was due to its being used to track down runaway slaves. Its lugubrious expression comes from the heavy jowls, which make the lower lids hang to give a bloodshot look to the eyes.

The bloodhounds have the most remarkable scenting ability of any dog and are able to track lost people through crowded city streets where the scent is weeks old and, in one case, even finding a criminal who was submerged in the middle of a lake, using a straw as a snorkel! The bloodhound makes a wonderful pet but is hard to recall when it gets on a scent. It can easily be hurt so use a soft voice for control. Unfortunately, bloodhounds do not have a long life span.

*Height*   Up to 69 cm.
*Weight*   Up to 50 kg.
*Colour*   Black and tan, liver and tan or red.

**Borzoi**   This sight hound from Russia was favoured by the royal courts. They valued this type of hound for working in the open so that the kings and courtiers could relish the gore at close quarters. It is aloof and does not like children. Sadly, it is often a fashion accessory.

*Height*   Up to 74 cm.
*Colour*   All colours.

**Dachshund**   Dachshunds were badger hounds in their native Germany and ideally built for the job, with feet like spades and good heavy shoulders. Their long back and their short legs gave them the right shape to dig into burrows. They are now bred much finer but still retain a curious desire to sleep at the bottom of beds under the covers. One of ours crawled down the centre of a rolled-up carpet and accidentally got sent to the dry-cleaners.

Owners are startled when their lazy lounge-lizard 'mother's darling' visits the country and goes mad catching rabbits! One owner hotly denied that her 'Dachsy' had killed a baby chook even as it looked her in the eye and hiccupped with the tell-tale yellow feathers hanging from the side of its mouth.

They bark at the slightest thing, and sound much bigger than they are! Although obstinate and not easy to train, they have enough personality to get away with it. They come in mini and standard sizes and are wire, smooth or long haired. Some are nervy. The type is also subject to diabetes and to slipped discs, due to the long back.

*Weight*   Standard: up to 12 kg; miniature: 4.5 kg.
*Colour*   All plain colours; a white spot on the chest is permitted.

**Deerhound** Woodcuts dated around 1560 show this dog to be much as it is today – rather like a shaggy greyhound from which it is descended. They are the most gentle house dogs, having for centuries lived inside feudal castles, lying by the hearth next to their dram-swigging masters. Depicted so often in ancient tapestries and paintings, the deerhound seems to add an exotic historic touch to its surroundings, wherever it may be.

They are wonderful with people and, incredibly enough, are an adaptable town dog. In the wilds of Scotland, however, their rather mincing gait suddenly transforms into enormous leaps and bounds at great speeds; when aroused they are ruthless killers of game, totally in contrast with their sweet and gentle nature with people.

*Height* Minimum 76 cm.
*Weight* About 45 kg.
*Colour* Dark blue-grey, darker and lighter greys or brindles and yellows, sandy reds or red fawns with black points.

**English Foxhound; American Foxhound; Harrier** The English and American foxhounds do not make suitable pets because they are very much members of a dog pack and tend to be too lively and destructive. The same is true for the harrier, a smaller hound that hunts the wild hare. The American foxhound is not a recognised breed in Australia.

*Height* Harrier: up to 53 cm.

**Greyhound** 'A Greyhund shud be heded lyke a Snake, and necked lyke a Drake, foted lyke a Kat, syded lyke a Bream. Chyned lyke a Beme.' So advises the book of St Albans, dated 1486. The greyhound is a very bright, trainable, gentle dog that makes the most delightful pet, so well behaved a child can handle it. Of course, the killer instinct is still there. It is a tragedy that its fate is invariably that of being destroyed because it did not run fast enough for its commercially minded owners who have had it put down with tears in their eyes because they could not afford a dog that did not pay its way – an extraordinary situation existing in the so-called name of sport.

I would recommend that more people give a home to a greyhound that did not make it in the racing game. I once sent a pensioner couple with their 18-year-old greyhound to a veterinary colleague who was a greyhound specialist. You should have seen the surprised looks on the faces of the other greyhound owners in his waiting room. This greyhound was exceptionally well loved and cared for, and she was so placid that she used to sleep on the sofa with the cat. Please spare some kindness for the too often cruelly treated greyhound.

*Height* Up to 76 cm.
*Colour* Black, white, red, blue, fawn, fallow or brindle, or any of these colours broken with white.

**Hamiltonstovare** This breed is a cross between the English foxhound and the best German hounds and is named after the founder of the breed Count Hamilton. It is the most popular hunting dog in Sweden today but does not make a suitable household pet.
*Height* Up to 58.5 cm.
*Colour* Tri-colour (black, tan and white).

**Ibizan and Pharaoh Hounds** Both the prick-eared Ibizan hound, which possesses the wilfulness of the hounds but is affectionate to its owner, and the Pharaoh hound, which is wary of strangers and totally unsuited to city life, are ancient breeds that hunt by sight and scent. Egyptian sculptures, depicting the god of Anubis, are the spitting images of these dogs that have obviously been around a very long time.
*Height* Ibizan: up to 74 cm; Pharaoh: ideally 56 cm.
*Colour* Ibizan: white, chestnut or lion; Pharaoh: tan or rich tan with white markings.

**Irish Wolfhound** Admired by Romans and given as gifts from kings, these dogs have attracted abundant legends. The story goes that an Irish hero, Fionn mac Cumall, had an aunt who was turned into a hound by an enemy. Cumall turned her back into human form again but was unable to do the same for her twins to which she gave birth while under the spell. These twins were the first pair of wolfhounds!
Wolfhounds are enormous dogs, bigger than the deerhound, and described, as long ago as 1698, as 'quiet as lambs' with people.
*Height* Up to 86 cm.
*Weight* 54.5 kg (minimum).
*Colour* Grey, brindle, red, black, pure white, fawn, wheaten or steel-grey.

**Otterhound** The otterhound's origin is somewhat obscure. It is an extremely old breed and was widely used for otter hunting in the time of King John, Henry II and Elizabeth. These hounds were kept by monks to guard fish ponds against otters. The breed would be extinct, as otter hunting is outlawed, but for a few devotees who kept the breed going. These hounds are affectionate. They have a shaggy coat.
*Height* Up to 68.5 cm.
*Weight* Up to 52.2 kg.
*Colour* All recognised hound colours but grizzly, not sharply demarked.

**Petit Basset Griffon Vendeen** This is one of the smaller French basset hounds and has a shaggy coat. It is an excellent hunter in dense cover, and an affectionate pet. When 'giving tongue', that is baying or barking, it strikes dread in the intruder! It needs plenty of exercise.
*Height* Up to 38 cm.
*Colour* White with any combination of lemon, orange, tri-colour (black, white and tan) or grizzle markings.

**Rhodesian Ridgeback** A primitive rock carving in Rhodesia shows dogs with a ridge of hair growing the wrong way round down their backs. It depicts a scene of the burial preparations for a famous Hottentot chief. These highly prized hunting dogs were in Africa long before the white man, and were probably descended from the Phu Quoc from the Siamese Gulf – the only other breed with this curious hair growth.

In modern Africa they are popular as guard dogs, excellent hunting dogs and reliable baby-sitters for children. Once they were used to hunt the lion, a most formidable foe; while they actually did not attack the lions, they made fighting gestures to distract the quarry so the shooter could approach stealthily – still pretty dangerous work for a dog!

The ridgeback, in rare cases, has an inherited defect: a small tract on the ridge which is subject to infection. A lovely dog who will settle down very comfortably on your lounge with the cat, the ridgeback has a great temperament but can be a little hard to train as it has a very short attention span. Sounds like a lot of children I know! They are also a large breed. One of my patients, Baza, once stood on a stranger's toe by mistake, and the afflicted party tried to sue Baza's owner – just one of the hazards of owning a large and heavy pet.
*Height* Up to 67 cm.
*Weight* Up to 36.3 kg.
*Colour* Light wheaten to red wheaten.

**Saluki** Often known as the gazelle hound, the saluki is a very ancient hound of royal lineage from Persia. These sight hounds do not bowl over strangers with friendliness, as do some of the gun dogs, but they do form very strong attachments to their owners.
*Height* Up to 71 cm.
*Colour* White, cream, fawn, golden red, grizzle, silver grizzle, deer grizzle, tri-colour (white, black and tan), black and tan and variations of these colours.

**Sloughi** This is the rarest of the sight hounds, cousin to the greyhound and hunter of the gazelle in the East. Although safe with children, it has strong hunting instincts. It is known by the Arabs as Elhor the aristocrat.

*Height*   Up to 76 cm.
*Colour*   Sandy, shades of fawn, may have black mask or saddle, also off-white, brindle, or black with tan and brindle.

**Spitz**   In Scandinavia there are a number of spitz dogs said to be descended from the northern wolf, with double coat, thick curled tail and prick ears. They include the powerful **elkhound**, which is capable of bringing down a 455-kg elk but makes a friendly and intelligent pet, and the smaller **Finnish spitz**, a hunter that is noisy, active and friendly.
*Height*   Elkhound: 52 cm; Finnish spitz: up to 50 cm.
*Weight*   Elkhound: about 23 kg; Finnish spitz: up to 16 kg.
*Colour*   Elkhound: grey; Finnish spitz: reddish brown or red-gold on back, white stripes on breast.

**Whippet**   Once known as the 'poor man's greyhound', the whippet was used by the workers in the North of England for weekend racing and as the ideal house pet during the week. Sadly, these dogs tend to get heart trouble. Also, the gentle whippet can often be the victim of a surprise attack from another dog because it runs with such speed that it will often enter another dog's territory too quickly to go through the doggy ritual of deciding who is top dog. One patient of mine comes in regularly to be stitched up and yet is not an aggressive dog. Silk-like skin and short hair make for a very clean house dog, although the whippet is hard to teach to recall.
*Height*   Up to 51 cm.
*Colour*   Any colour or mix of colours.

# THE WORKING DOGS

The natural basic instincts of these dogs have been specially developed so that they can do important jobs of work. Without their jobs to perform, many of these dogs as pets sublimate their natural instincts, as do kelpies for example, by chasing cars while border collies round up anything they can find. The natural herder let loose in the country can, if not trained for the job, run amok in a flock of sheep, creating havoc. The worker dogs are herders, haulers or guards.

**Anatolian Shepherd, or Karabash**   This one-person dog, intelligent and loyal, is found across the Anatolian plateau of Turkey to Afghanistan and guards rather than herds flocks. It is an ancient breed descended from dogs of Babylonian times. In its native country it often has cropped ears, and wears a huge spiked collar to help fight

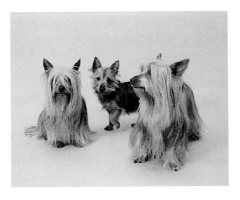

*Australian silky terrier*

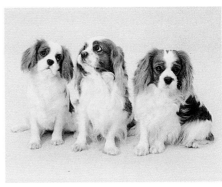

*Cavalier King Charles spaniel*

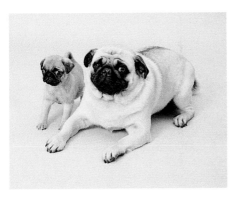

*Pug*

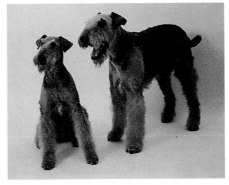

*Airedale terrier*

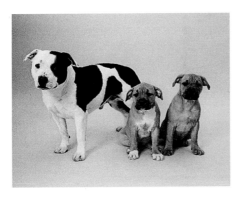

*Staffordshire bull terrier*

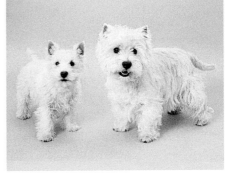

*West Highland white terrier*

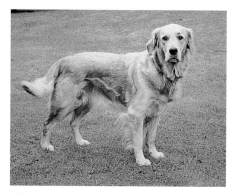

*Golden retriever*

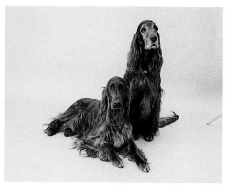

*Irish setter*

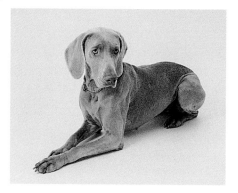

*Weimaraner*

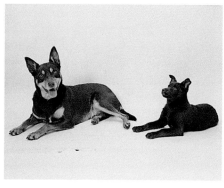

*Australian kelpie*

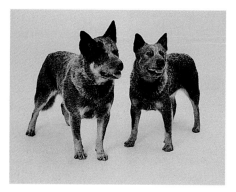

*Australian cattle dog*

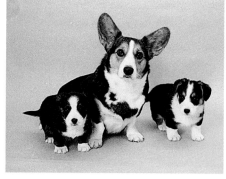

*Welsh corgi (Cardigan)*

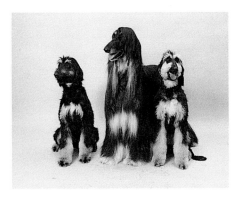

*Afghan hound*

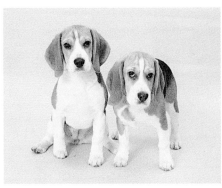

*Beagle*

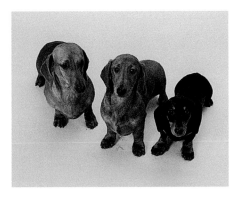

*Dachshund (smooth-haired)*

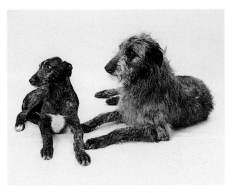

*Deerhound*

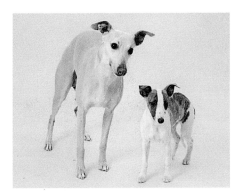

*Whippet*

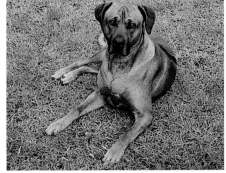

*Rhodesian ridgeback*

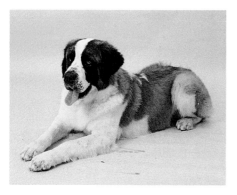

*St Bernard*

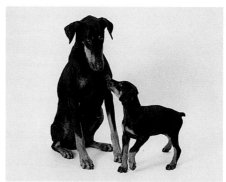

*Dobermann*

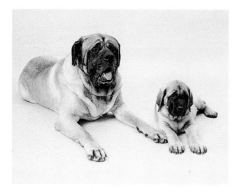

*Mastiff*

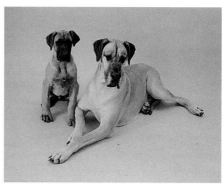

*Great Dane*

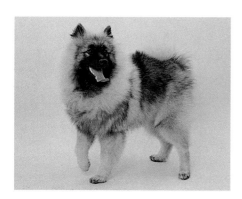

*Keeshond*

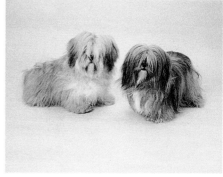

*Lhasa apso*

predators. These dogs have, as a group, inborn ambush tactics. They are not highly suitable as pets because of their need for freedom.
*Height*  Up to 81 cm.
*Weight*  Up to 64 kg.
*Colour*  All shades of fawn, maybe with white socks and chest blaze, and black mask.

**Australian Cattle Dog**  Australia has two working dogs whose fame is spreading worldwide: the cattle dog and the kelpie. The cattle dog could not be more different from the kelpie. It derived from the crossing of blue smooth-coated collies, or 'merles', with kelpies with a dash of Dalmatian (probably where the inherited deafness in some dogs comes from) and a splash of dingo thrown in. This cattle-drover's dog or 'heeler' has great initiative, working by silently nipping at the heels of cattle. This tendency can cause some dogs to bite unpredictably with a nip on the ankle.
*Height*  Up to 51 cm.
*Weight*  Up to 15.9 kg.
*Colour*  Blue: blue-mottled or speckled; red: red-speckled all over.

**Australian Kelpie**  The kelpie got its name from a sheepdog that won the trials at Forbes in New South Wales in 1872. The word 'kelpie' refers to a water spirit that lures travellers off their pathway on the misty moorland!

Kelpies were all bred from three pairs of black and tan, smooth-coated working collies from Scotland and, even in our machine-driven age, they are still irreplaceable by anything mechanical: they do the work of three men. Out on the sheep station, you see them running across the backs of a mob of sheep, able to work well out of sight of their owners.

The kelpie is not a suitable town dog, although very loving and permissive, because its ability to work long hours, tough conditions and high temperatures has little outlet in the city; it can only sub-limate its instincts by chasing cars. The kelpie is easily trained, being very anxious to please by nature. It will roll on its back in contrition if you raise your voice, then leap up and cover you with kisses when you become forgiving.
*Height*  Up to 51 cm.
*Weight*  Up to about 13.6 kg.
*Colour*  Black, black and tan, red, red and tan, fawn, chocolate or smoky blue.

Many Australian crossbreeds are mixtures of the cattle dog and the kelpie and become stray dogs. Although a particular crossbreed may look either more kelpie or more cattle dog, you have to observe its behaviour to determine its temperament. Many of these crossbreeds make excellent pets in the middle-range size, but remember they need plenty of exercise in the city and must be under control in the country because the worker dog, not trained to work, can become a worrier of livestock.

**Belgian Shepherd** This breed is divided into four categories, all of which make excellent guards and herders. There are the long-coated Groenendael and Tervueren, the smooth-coated Malinois and the wire-coated Laekenois. Like the German shepherd, the Belgian needs the right training to get good results.
*Height* Up to 66 cm.
*Colour* Laekenois, Tervueren and Malinois: all shades of red, fawn, grey with overlay; Groenendael: black or black with limited white.

**Bouvier des Flandres** This type was bred from a number of Belgian working dogs, resulting in a dog used as a herder and for draught purposes. It is a devoted one-person dog with a strong guarding ability and needs lots of exercise. It has a rough ill-kempt appearance, and is not very suitable for the city.
*Height* Up to 68 cm.
*Weight* Up to 40 kg.
*Colour* From fawn to black, including brindle.

**Briard** This is a well-known French sheepdog. The name is easy to re-member if you like brie cheese, because that is the French cheese-producing region from which these dogs come. In the church at Mont-didier is a shield carved on stone showing a dog's head – that of a Briard. It commemorates the dog owner Sir Aubry Montdidier, who was assassinated in 1371 and whose killer was hunted down by his dog. To see justice done, the King ordered a battle between the killer and Sir Aubry's dog on the Isle of Notre Dame. The dog won the battle and the killer was duly executed. Despite this grisly story, the Briard, believe it or not, is a shaggy, friendly dog but does need plenty of exercise.
*Height* Up to 68 cm.
*Colour* All black or black with white hairs scattered through; all shades of fawn.

**German Shepherd Dog** This breed evokes very strong public feeling for and against dogs. It is, perhaps, the most intelligent of all breeds and, like an exceptionally gifted child, will go wrong if it has a life that does not challenge its intellectual potential. Because of the dog's deserved reputation for excellent guarding instincts, many unsuitable people buy them as guards and leave them chained to a clothes hoist all day. This degree of frustration for an active dog could turn it savage, noisy and destructive – as it could many other dogs.

The German shepherd, treated as it should be however, is one of the most reliable dogs available. Popularity of course means that some have been bred with undesirable temperaments and some have hip dysplasia, so you should only buy from stock that is registered free from hip dysplasia.

German shepherd dogs were unknown in the United Kingdom before the First World War, and then the British were stunned by their incredible feats in the German army. Some were brought back to Britain after the war where for many years they were known as Alsatians. Used as herders, they came from the French border province of Alsace-Lorraine where there was an understandably strong prejudice against anything bearing a German name.

Nowadays, they are guide dogs for the blind in the United States and used extensively as police and guard dogs all over the world. Many countries have special training classes for German shepherd dogs so make enquiries through your local kennel control body.

*Height*   Ideal 62.5 cm.
*Colour*   Black or black saddle with tan; all black, all grey or with lighter or brown markings.

**Hungarian Puli**   Europe of course abounds with working dogs but among the most popular in other parts of the world is the puli. This ancient Magyar herding dog of Hungary sports a coat of Rastafarian dreadlocks that would be the envy of every West Indian in the Portobello Road in London. At least you do not have to do anything to frizz up these tightly curled ringlets – they just happen! I would have thought, however, that this coat would be a playground for fleas in a hot climate. Talking to one breeder of pulis in Sydney, I was told that they completely doused the house with insecticide once a week. I wondered who would be moving out first – the breeder or the dog!

Pulis are quite willful dogs and, to stop them roaming off on the Hungarian plains, they used to wear a heavy iron loop around the neck that banged on their knees if they tried to make a move.

*Height*   Up to 44 cm.
*Weight*   Up to 15 kg.
*Colour*   Black, rusty black, white and various shades of grey and apricot.

**Kuvasz**   This is a large, white Hungarian dog not unlike the Pyrenean mountain dog and, although it has herding ability, is mainly used as a guard, popular in this role since the fifteenth century when King Matthias was never without one on his large estates. These dogs

probably originated in Tibet and came to Hungary with the Turks. They need a daily brush.
*Colour*  White.

**Maremma Sheepdog**  This sheepdog is probably of Magyar origin and believed to have been recorded 2000 years ago. This large dog of the Tuscan farmers of Italy is a guard and herder of sheep. It is extremely strong-willed and hard to train, and fierce when guarding home or child. This dog is a free spirit, not to be confined as a house pet.
*Height*  Up to 73 cm.
*Weight*  Up to 45 kg.
*Colour*  White.

**Norwegian Buhund**  This breed is both a herder and guard dog and a good family dog of the northern spitz variety. It is sharp but friendly and good with children.
*Height*  Up to 45 cm.
*Weight*  In proportion to size.
*Colour*  Wheaten, black, medium red or wolf-sable.

**Old English Sheepdog**  Often known as the bobtail, as some are born with a stumpy tail, they otherwise have long tails that are unfortunately docked. You must discipline yourself to give this dog once a week a thorough grooming session with a steel comb and a daily brushing. Knots easily gather around the feet so that they look like snowballs.

Although considered English, the origin of these sheepdogs is disputable; they may have come from the Briard crossed with the Russian Owtscharka, which is related in turn to Hungarian sheepdogs. But then I bet you didn't know that the famous 'English' actor, Leslie Howard, was a Hungarian too!

Easily trained but beware – many have hip dysplasia.
*Height*  61 cm.
*Colour*  All shades of grey, grizzle or blue.

**Polish Lowland Sheepdog**  Introduced to Poland in the fourth and fifth century, this breed looks something like the Old English sheepdog. It is intelligent and good natured.
*Height*  Up to 52 cm.
*Colour*  All colours.

**Pumi**  A much more recent breed than the Hungarian puli, the pumi is a herder of cattle and swine as well as a police dog. It has an untidy coat but does not boast the dreadlocks or ropey ringlets of the puli. This breed is not recognised in Australia.

**Shetland Sheepdog**   Also known as a sheltie, this dog is like a rough collie in miniature. It is an excellent family pet but often very wary of strangers. These dogs came from the Shetland Isles off the north coast of Scotland. They can easily be trained.
*Height*   Up to 37 cm.
*Colour*   Sable: clear or shaded, any colour from pale gold to deep mahogany; tri-colour: intense black on body with rich tan markings; blue merle: clear silvery blue, splashed and marbled with black; black and white or black and tan.

**Stumpy-tailed Cattle Dog**   This cattle dog is descended from the same line as the Australian cattle dog, but came from a line born with a bobtail. It originated with a drover named Timmins and is referred to as a Timmins' biter.
*Height*   Up to 51 cm.
*Colour*   Red-speckled, blue or blue-mottled.

**Swedish Vallhund**   This dog looks like a corgi, and the million-dollar question is: did the Vikings pinch it from Wales, or did they take it to the United Kingdom? These are great cattle dogs and pets and although, like the corgi, they will adapt to little exercise, if they don't have enough they will become overweight.
*Height*   Up to 35 cm.
*Weight*   Up to 15.9 kg.
*Colour*   Steel-grey, greyish brown, greyish yellow, reddish yellow or reddish brown.

## The Collies

Once upon a time, before England and Scotland were industrialised, sheep needed looking after as they roamed free and were not confined to fields. This is still true in parts of Scotland and Wales and on the moors in the west of England but in those pre-industrial days there were many working collies with great reputations. They would drop to the ground instantly as if shot through the head at the smallest hiss signal from the shepherd. Nowadays, it is only the border collie that remains the efficient worker and the others of this breed have become popular as pets.

**Bearded Collie**   This collie looks a bit like an Old English sheepdog and was probably partly descended from some Polish sheepdog with a bit of Hungarian blood thrown in, but the origins are disputable. It is popular in the show ring and as a pet. It is a little soft to be a

good worker now, although it retains its herding instincts. It makes a good house pet.
*Height*  Up to 56 cm.
*Colour*  Slate grey, reddish fawn, black, blue, all shades of grey, brown or sandy with or without white markings.

**Border Collie**  The star of the sheepdogs and famous throughout the world, this dog will round up anything! It is not ideally suited to the city, although it can make a good pet.

Mindy was such a dog. No longer wanted for breeding, she was about to be shot after having given birth to the litter she was carrying. A horrified visitor to Mindy's owners' farm made off with her and took her to a vet friend of mine who lived in the Australian bush. Here she was desexed and treated for heartworm, as her previous owners had never bothered to have her on preventative treatment. She was then given a home in the heart of Sydney with the vet's mother. Now she happily rounds up low-flying swallows in the park.

Border collies came from the border and lowland areas of Scotland and England. Speed, agility and endurance are the name of the game with these dogs. They tolerate the harshness of the Australian climate really well, in spite of their background, as the long coat gives protection in the heat.
*Height*  Up to 53 cm.
*Colour*  Black and white mainly, but can also be blue, chocolate, red or black and tan, all with white markings.

**Rough Collie**  The rough collie is best known as the film star 'Lassie'. The type was probably originally descended from Icelandic dogs and got its name because it used to guard the black-faced and black-legged sheep known as colleys in Scotland. The cascading coat needs a lot of care: the vacuum cleaner can come in handy to clean off dry mud. The now-exaggerated long nose loves sniffing in embarrassing spots and can also get a condition called 'collie nose'. These collies are good with children. Sadly, because of television popularity, too many were bought for the wrong reasons and often ended up as strays.
*Height*  Up to 61 cm.
*Weight*  Up to 29.5 kg.
*Colour*  Sable and white, tri-colour (black, tan and white) or blue merle.

**Smooth Collie**  This dog is just like the rough collie except for its coat. If you choose one of these dogs in preference to the rough, you will not have all that work looking after the coat, but then hair has always been such a scene stealer!

*Height*  Up to 61 cm.
*Weight*  Up to 29.5 kg.
*Colour*  Sable and white, tri-colour (black, tan and white) and blue merle.


## The Welsh Corgis

There is now a sharp drop in size to the corgis. This Welsh cattle dog is near to the ground for a very good reason: when it goes in to heel or nip at the heels of the cattle, a smart backward kick just sails over its head. Corgis have been working cattle since the Doomsday book appeared in the eleventh century in south Wales.

Although only weighing up to 12 kg, corgis are a handful in terms of personality. Being a worker, they need quite a bit of exercise or they will become rather square.

They are often a popular pet for the elderly but I think they are far more suitable as a family dog. They are a bit too busy for elderly people and may trip them up. Also, the tendency to nip must be strictly discouraged. I'd go for the **Cardigan corgi**. It has a long tail and is a little quieter than most but be aware of the inherited condition of progressive retinal atrophy – blindness due to degeneration of the retina. Corgis tend to get skin trouble in the hot weather, especially in a climate such as Australia.

*Height*  Ideal 30 cm.
*Weight*  Up to 12 kg.
*Colour*  Any colour with or without white markings.

**Pembroke Corgi**  This corgi, which is tailless, is very popular because of its connection with the royal family. When I was a student, I was asked to scale a corgi's teeth. When I had finished, the Professor said 'Now you will be able to put "By Royal Appointment" after your name!'. I am not sure the royal family would have appreciated either his sense of humour or my scaling their dog's teeth!
*Height*  Up to 30.5 cm.
*Weight*  Up to 12 kg.
*Colour*  Red, sable, fawn or black and tan.


# THE UTILITY DOGS

**Akita**  A Japanese breed and one of the most important in that country, the akita was once only owned by royalty in mediaeval Japan where a special language was devised both to speak to and about them.

The handlers also wore an elaborate costume. These dogs are essentially hunters of the spitz variety and look rather like a long-legged chow. The breed has become an affectionate family pet and guardian of children.
*Height*   Up to 71 cm.
*Colour*   Any colour.

**Alaskan Malamute**   This serious sledge dog of Alaska was probably the breed most famous in Jack London's novels about those frozen wastelands. The lighter Siberian husky was mostly used by the Russians in their cross-country treks to charter the Siberian coast because a lighter dog could cover a bigger distance in the shortest time. Today, however, the Malamute is used for long-distance sled racing; six dogs pull 364 kg up to 16 kilometres per hour for 64 or 80 kilometres per day, no mean task even for a 57-kg dog of solid build and flat feet for coping in the snow. Almond-eyed and wolf-like in appearance, the malamutes actually have a beautiful temperament and make a wonderful pet, although strong willed. Exercise is essential. A great deal of research has been done by vets on the stress-related problems of malamutes, caused by the rigours of racing. The Eskimo and Greenland varieties of this dog are other tough outdoor characters mainly confined to the Polar areas.
*Height*   Up to 71 cm.
*Weight*   Up to 57 kg.
*Colour*   From light grey through to black, or gold through red to liver, always with white on underbody.

**Bernese Mountain Dog**   This huge dog, of very amiable disposition, has for centuries been used for hauling. In fact, some dogs still pull along milk-carts in Switzerland. This breed is very placid and makes a good pet.
*Height*   Up to 70 cm.
*Colour*   Black, tan and white.

**Boxer**   A relatively new German breed, also derived from the mastiff and bulldog plus some other breeds, the boxer has turned out to be one of the most popular breeds in the world today. Boxers are real 'hams', notoriously boisterous and amiable and very smart to look at, in spite of the 'monkey face' appearance due to the undershot jaw.
*Height*   Up to 63 cm.
*Weight*   Up to 32 kg.
*Colour*   Fawn or brindle; white markings acceptable not exceeding one-third of ground colour.

**Bullmastiff**　This breed is a more recent development, coming from the mastiff and probably the bulldog. It has a great temperament and, though a good guard, was a favourite dog of gamekeepers at the end of the nineteenth century.
*Height*　Up to 68.5 cm.
*Weight*　Up to 59 kg.
*Colour*　Any shade of brindle, fawn or red.

**Dobermann**　This breed was developed in 1870 by Herr Dobermann in Germany, and is now one of the world's most popular dogs. Herr Dobermann was a tax collector and no doubt it was the reception he got on his tax-collecting rounds that stimulated him to breed a new dog for his own protection. This task was made easier by the fact that he was also the keeper of the local pound, which gave him plenty of stock from which to choose.

Excellent guard dogs used by the police and the army, their nature depends greatly upon the personality of the owner, provided that you have a reliable strain of dog. They can be incredibly sooky in the hands of some people and in the wrong hands can be aggressive. They make an excellent pet with proper direction and training.
*Height*　Up to 69 cm.
*Weight*　About 20.4 kg.
*Colour*　Definite black, brown, blue or fawn with rust-red markings.

**German Pinscher**　This medium-sized and short-coated breed is the origin of the Dobermann and miniature pinscher. It is a sporting dog, great ratter and watch dog.
*Height*　Up to 48 cm.
*Colour*　All solid colours from fawn to red in various shades, or black and blue with reddish tan markings.

**Komondor**　This larger herder from Hungary is claimed to have wiped out the wolf in that country! It has a corded white coat with small sections twisted to give the appearance of rope, just like the puli's coat.
*Height*　80 cm.
*Weight*　Up to 61 kg.
*Colour*　White.

**Leonberger**　Bred by Herrn Essig who wanted to evolve a dog that would look like the coat of arms of the town of Leonberger, this dog is said to be Newfoundland Pyrenean and St Bernard cross.
*Height*　Up to 80 cm.
*Colour*　Yellow to reddish brown, dark mask, some slight variations.

**Mastiff**  One of the first jobs performed by dogs of ancient times was that of guard, and of those guard dogs the oldest example is the mastiff. A Roman officer was stationed at Winchester in England, just after the Roman occupation, to collect the best specimens of mastiff to send to Rome, where they fought in the Colosseum. The breed is probably Asiatic in origin as similar dogs are depicted in the Assyrian gallery at the British Museum in artworks dating from the seventh century BC. Even earlier representations of the mastiff appear in Babylonian reliefs dating back as far as 2200 BC.

It is hard to breed dogs with good bone, that is good shape and strength, in this day and age, whereas the ancient model of mastiff possessed great physical perfection. An extract from a nineteenth-century book on dogs aptly describes its temperament: 'His courage does not exceed his temper and generosity. I have seen him down, with his paw, a terrier or cur, that has bitten him without offering further injury; he will permit the children to play with him and suffer all their little pranks without offence.' What a wonderful baby-sitter! It is sad that these gentle giants are so rarely seen these days; their temperament is so wonderful and they are such a magnificent, living part of our history.

*Height*  Up to 76 cm.
*Colour*  Apricot-fawn, silver-fawn or dark fawn-brindle.

**Neopolitan Mastiff**  This is an ancient breed from southern Italy, probably from the Roman Molossus, which looks incredibly fierce but is gentle and generally only attacks on command. It is a guard, police dog and tracker. The breed is not recognised in Australia.

*Height*  Up to 75 cm.
*Weight*  Up to 70 kg.
*Colour*  Black, lead, mouse-grey, streaked; may have small white spots on chest and tail.

**Newfoundland**  This breed is another great nanny and rescuer (but this time from water rather than snow). It was in Newfoundland in northeastern Canada that fishing fleets of other nations came to shelter from storms, bringing with them their dogs, such as Red Indian dogs and Basque sheepdogs, which probably mated with the local dogs to produce the Newfoundland. The nineteenth-century British painter Sir Edward Landseer made the black and white variety well known from his oil paintings, and this type now bears his name. They have a strong instinct to carry anything in the water to safety and one patient I was visiting promptly 'rescued' my surgery bag from my hand and carried it up the garden path.

*Height*  Up to 71 cm.

*Weight*   Up to 69 kg.
*Colour*   Dull jet black, chocolate or bronze or white with black markings.

**Portuguese Water Dog**   This ancient breed from the water dogs of Europe is poodle-like and clipped close on the hindquarters. It is a working member of the crew on the fishermen's boats on the Algarve coast of Portugal, guarding nets and even retrieving fish. This dog is suspicious of strangers. It is not a recognised breed in Australia.
*Height*   Up to 57 cm.
*Weight*   Up to 25 kg.
*Colour*   Black, white, various shades of brown, or black or brown combined with white.

**Pyrenean Mountain Dog**   This dog is huge and mainly white. Its ancestors, who guarded flocks against the wolves and sheep-thieves, probably got their fierceness from their even more remote Asiatic ancestors. Early types of this dog were used in battle as far back as Charlemagne, Hannibal and Alexander the Great.

This French working dog is comparatively rare in its own country now. Traditionally the double dew claws are left on the hind legs, probably to help them cope with snowy terrain. Although a great family dog, they can tend, being instinctively excellent guards, to take a piece out of a stranger. They eat a lot, shed white hair everywhere, but on the plus side they do not need a huge amount of exercise.
*Height*   71 cm.
*Weight*   Up to 50 kg.
*Colour*   Mainly white with patches of badger, wolf-grey or pale yellow.

**Rottweiler**   In the Middle Ages, the Rottweiler was a boar hunter; later, in the town of Rottweil in Germany, it became the butcher's drover dog, a handy companion when coming back from market with a bag full of money. A big, cloddy dog, it was recognised as a great guard and police dog just before the First World War.

If not exercised properly to keep its figure, the Rottweiler can become lazy in a hot climate whereas a dog with the reputation of a butcher's draught dog should be active and tough. Sadly, their popularity has meant that some unreliable strains have been bred from bad stock, but the odd rotten Rotty is more than compensated for by the many with a great temperament. This dog needs good training.
*Height*   Up to 69 cm.
*Colour*   Black and tan.

**St Bernard**   This is one of the giant super-nannies of the dog world –
Wendy's family in *Peter Pan* actually called their St Bernard 'Nanny'.
Fantastic with children, the sad part is that they do not live to a great
old age. Most people are familiar with them from the advertisement
that depicts a St Bernard with a barrel of brandy hanging around its
neck – a warming thought, being awoken from an impending frozen
death in the snow by a warm tongue and a cognac! Descending from
the Roman Molossus dogs, they were named after the St Bernhard
Hospice in the Swiss Alps where one hero called Barry notched up
40 snow rescues.

Poor bone is a problem, especially in the back legs. This dog is
renowned for drooling and also needs lots of space. It is expensive
to feed.
*Weight*   Up to about 90.8 kg.
*Colour*   Orange, mahogany brindle, red brindle, with white patches.

**Samoyed**   The Samoyed is the most popular of the sledge dogs. A
nomadic dog of the wandering Siberian tribes, it served as a hauling
dog and also guarded the flocks. Ceremonial garments were woven
from the combings of its thick double undercoat; some devoted
breeders still continue this practice. The Samoyed as a pet likes to
go 'walkabout', so see it gets plenty of exercise. It has flat feet like
snow shoes.
*Height*   Up to 56 cm.
*Colour*   Pure white, white and biscuit, cream, outer coat silver-tipped.

**Schnauzer**   This German dog was useful as a herder and later as a
guard of factories. Its temperament is essentially that of the terrier.
These dogs come in **giant**, **standard** and **miniature** sizes. The latter
is very popular as a pet, has a very strong will of its own and is apt
to run the family, but with great charm! All are good guard dogs.
*Height*   Giant: up to 70 cm; standard: ideal 48 cm; miniature: ideal
35.5 cm.
*Colour*   Pepper and salt on black.

**Shiba Inu**   This name means 'small dog' and the breed is the smallest
of the ancient hunting dogs of Japan, a typical spitz with double coat,
quite highly strung, cheerful and a good guard.
*Height*   Up to 39.5 cm.
*Colour*   Red, black, tan and black, and sometimes brindle; white
with red or grey tinge.

**Siberian Husky**   This breed is gaining in popularity as a pet and is
alert, intelligent, a good family member and sensitive to changes in
its environment.

*Height*   Up to 39.5 cm.
*Weight*   In proportion to size.
*Colour*   Red, black, black and tan or brindle; white with red or grey
tinge.

**Tibetan Mastiff**   Probably descended from the Roman Molossus like
other mastiffs, this large guard dog, looking more like a St Bernard
than a mastiff, originated in the foothills of the Himalayas and Central
Asia. It is a guard and herder and not as fierce as other mastiffs, a
welcome fact to know if you are trekking in Nepal! It has a curly tail
like smaller Tibetan breeds.
*Height*   Up to 66 cm.
*Colour*   Black, black and tan, brown, and various shades of gold or grey.

# THE NON-SPORTING DOGS

**Boston Terrier**   This is the all-American dog but, like the human in-
habitants of that country, came originally from a mixture of overseas
types, mainly bulldog and English terrier with a bit of French bulldog
thrown in. The result is an erect-eared, screw-tailed, squashed-faced
little character who comes in light, middle and heavyweight sizes.
Makes a delightful house dog.
*Weight*   Up to 11.4 kg.
*Colour*   Brindle with white markings.

**British Bulldog**   This Churchillian character was bred to bait the bull,
a barbaric sport popular in the time of Henry VIII and not abolished
by British parliament until 1835. It was bred with shoulders low to
the ground so that it could come at the bull below the level of his
horns and seize and hold onto its nose. The game bull was one that
had been baited before; the poor brute had then learnt to paw a hole
in the ground to bury his nose for protection and then to toss the
dog often as high as 10 metres into the air. The dog's nose was set
almost on top of its face so that it could breathe while pinning the
bull. Modern breeders exaggerated these physical characteristics so
that the modern bulldog could not even bait a mouse!

They are now loveable characters but still suffer from breathing
problems because of their tortuous nasal passages. Folds on the face
may need lubricating. They do not live to a great age nor do they appreciate a hot climate.
*Weight*   Up to 25 kg.
*Colour*   Whole or smut (whole colour with black mask or muzzle);
whole colours can be brindle, red, fawn or fallow.

**Chow Chow**   This dog has the legendary inscrutability of the East and has been known in China for over two thousand years. The name comes from the pidgin English for mixed food sold in China, which is unpleasantly appropriate because the chow chow was historically valued for its meat and for its skins for garments. One might well then forgive this dog its haughty demeanour and lack of friendliness to all people except its owner, to whom it will be totally devoted. A chow chow is a loner. It is not easy to train and if you do not pack-leader it then it will soon pack-leader you! The thick double coat, curly tail and prick ears are typical features of the spitz dogs of the northern hemisphere. They are prone to skin troubles in a hot climate. A curious feature of the chow chow is its straight back legs and blue tongue. A shorter-coated variety is popular in Hong Kong and is used for guarding the waterfronts.
*Height*   Up to 56 cm.
*Colour*   Whole coloured black, red, blue, fawn, cream or white.

**Dalmatian**   This white dog with black or liver spots, known as the 'plum pudding' dog, was historically reputed to have been a guard dog along the coast of Dalmatia and Croatia against the invasion of the Turks. Later it became a highly fashionable carriage dog in nineteenth-century England, living in the stables with the horses and accompanying carriages by running alongside, sometimes right under the back axle.

In 1851 there was one famous Dalmatian who did the London to Brighton run of about 72 miles (115 kilometres) often on seven successive days. One day, however, he fell to his death under the wheels of the carriage. His stuffed remains were proudly preserved under glass in a pub in the Edgeware Road in London.

A very clean house dog with plenty of endurance and intelligence, the Dalmatian may suffer from an inherited tendency to kidney stones and deafness.
*Height*   Up to 61 cm.
*Colour*   Pure white with either dense black spots or liver-brown spots.

**French Bulldog**   This breed is claimed to have originated with the Doge de Bordeaux and, although it is certainly a wholly French product, probably came originally from small English bulldogs. It has a squashed face, erect rounded ears and a delightful personality; it has an outgoing manner but can sulk if it wants. The folds on its face can become sore and need lubricating.
*Weight*   Up to 12.7 kg.
*Colour*   Brindle, pied or fawn.

**German Spitz**   This is another breed of spitz.
*Height*   Klein (small): up to 28 cm; mittel (medium-sized): up to 35.5 cm.
*Colour*   All varieties of colour and markings allowed.

**Great Dane**   Hundreds of 'Hamlets' abound in the Great Dane world, named of course after the famous Danish prince, but in fact this dog probably came from the Molossus hounds of Roman times in Great Britain. In late nineteenth-century Germany, Bismarck crossed the mastiffs from the south of Germany with the northern Great Dane to produce a type very much like the Great Dane of today.
   The Great Dane is a disaster if bought as a status symbol dog; in such cases the owners are often nervous with the dog – and such a lot of dog – and without the right direction there will be a lot of problems. They do not live to a grand old age, and, like all giant breeds, are subject to arthritis if they are constantly pounding the pavement with their jogger owners. Fortunately, they usually get on well with other dogs.
*Height*   Up to 76 cm.
*Weight*   Up to 54 kg.
*Colour*   Black; brindle: lightest buff to deepest orange with black stripes; fawn: lightest buff to deepest orange; blue: light grey to deep slate; harlequin: pure white with black or blue patches.

**Japanese Spitz**   A herder related to the Norrbotten Swedish spitz dog, this lovely, intelligent one-person dog can adapt to city life if exercised enough.
*Height*   Up to 36 cm.
*Colour*   Pure white.

**Keeshond**   Another spitz breed, probably descended from the German wolf spitz, the keeshond is also known as the Dutch barge dog; it was a popular dog on the waterways of Holland and is therefore able to cope with a fairly confined space. The dog is quite vocal, naturally making an excellent guard dog. He was probably named after Kees de Witt or Kees de Gyselaer, seventeenth- and eighteenth-century Dutch patriots, or from the Keezen, the word for 'rabble', which referred to the people's party opposed to the House of Orange. These dogs may suffer from inherited epilepsy.
*Height*   Up to 45.7 cm.
*Colour*   A mixture of grey and black.

**Llasa Apso**   It is hard to reconcile the appearance of this merry, amusing little dog, sporting its cascades of long hair (that make it difficult to tell which end is which), with its dignified background as a holy dog in the monasteries of Tibet. It was firmly believed by the Tibetan monks that the souls of the high priests, or lamas, entered the bodies of the dogs when the priests died. It may be that the great respect that these dogs commanded accounts for trying to get away with murder, because the apso can certainly sometimes resent an owner's authority. It strides out, when walking, with the gait of a trotter and is very sturdy.

This is not surprising when you consider that they were presented by the lamas of Tibet to the Empress of China and made their way to the Imperial Palace, accompanying the monks' caravans on foot.

*Height*   Up to 25.4 cm.

*Colour*   Golden, sandy, honey, dark grizzle, slate, smoke-coloured, parti-colour (partly one colour, partly another or other colours), black, white or brown.

**Poodle**   It is surprising the number of people there are who do not want to own a poodle because they find the traditional hair-cut ridiculous. The poodle has always been associated with the fashion world, suffering all sorts of indignities like being dyed the colour purple. I have seen many a fur-coated lady of the night in London, soliciting while accompanied by her poodle as a fashion accessory.

This dog's background however is sporting and the name comes from the German word *pudeln* meaning 'to splash in water'. The coat, cut into pom-poms over the joints, was to protect it when retrieving game in freezing cold water and the bow on the head and pom-pom on the tail enabled the shooter to easily distinguish it from a duck at long distance. The long hair over the chest was to protect the lungs. Special poodle barbers on the banks of the Seine during the reign of Louis XVI cut their coats into intricate patterns such as lovers' knots. They were also popular dogs in the French circus as they are particularly easy to train.

Their temperament has always been described as 'gay'. Nowadays we have had to replace this description with such phrases as 'full of high spirits', which does not quite fit the bill like the old meaning of the word 'gay'.

Poodles come in standard, miniature and toy sizes and you can have a sensible 'Dutch' hairdo instead of the traditional one. These dogs are excellent for children who suffer from allergies as they do not shed hair like other dogs.

*Height*   Standard: above 38 cm; miniature: under 38 cm; toys: under 28 cm.

*Colour*   All solid colours.

**Schipperke** Another spitz breed but with a docked tail, the schipperke was a barge dog in Belgium. It is very active and inquisitive and makes an excellent guard dog.
*Weight* Up to 7.3 kg.
*Colour* Usually black, but also other whole colours.

**Shar-pei** A dog that has been included in the Guinness Book of Records as the world's rarest has sadly got a pretty rough deal. Status-symbol seekers create a market for unscrupulous breeders, these charge ludicrous prices for dogs that are so inbred they suffer from a long list of inherited defects.

Dating back to the Han Dynasty, the shar-pei became known much later as the 'Chinese fighting dog' when it was used for dog fights by the fishermen on the wharves. As the shar-pei is naturally an affectionate, intelligent dog, good with children, it is not hard to believe the rumour that they were given drugs to make them aggressive for such fighting. Due to a high 'dog tax' that made it virtually impossible to own a dog, the breed was almost extinct in China by 1947 as most were being used for food.

Shar-peis are covered in wrinkles with a curved tail and squashed face. Specially bred for fighting, the multiple folds of skin made it hard for another dog to get a hold, earning it the name 'the dog God forgot to inflate'. They are also nicknamed 'ruffle pups'. If the stiff, short hair is too short where the skin folds, the hair will prick the dog's own skin causing bad dermatological problems. Entropion (or lids rolling in on the eye), breathing and breeding problems and sometimes a poor immune system can occur. In spite of this, you can get very healthy specimens. They are delightful dogs. If you fancy one, make sure you research your breeders as there are some who do take a caring and not a commercial attitude to their dogs.
*Height* Up to 51 cm.
*Weight* Up to 22.7 kg.
*Colour* Solid colours: black, red, light or dark shades of fawn or cream.

**Shih Tzu** The apso was crossed with the Chinese Pekingese to make the shih tzu, a similarly revered dog with an equally appealing personality.
*Height* Up to 26.7 cm.
*Weight* Up to 8.2 kg.
*Colour* All colours.

**Tibetan Terrier** This breed is the worker of this group, being a herder and guard in the rural areas. It is a more rough-and-tumble version of the other Tibetan breeds and looks not unlike a miniature Old

English sheepdog. The feet, unlike those of other terriers, are flat to cope with rough mountain terrain. They are typically active terriers.
*Height* Up to 40.6 cm.
*Colour* White, golden, cream, grey or smoke-coloured, or black.

**Tibetan Spaniel** This spaniel was also part of the monastic life of Tibet; it would turn the prayer wheels. Its efforts brought the prayers nearer to heaven with every turn of the wheel, which contained parchment scrolls. Tibetan spaniels are temperamentally similar to the other small oriental breeds and their devotees very much resent them being mistaken for toy breeds. Although breeds such as these are distinctive in the Western world, in Nepal and Tibet such dogs are everywhere, with ill-kept coats and often treated very much as part of the family. As I passed a stone house in a village in a remote part of Nepal, I spotted a family seated in a circle on the floor having a meal. One member of this intimate circle was the family dog.
*Height* About 25 cm.
*Weight* Up to 8 kg.
*Colour* All colours.

PART II

# Settling In

# 4

# Puppy Comes Home

## TRAVEL ARRANGEMENTS: THE JOURNEY HOME

Arrange with the breeder for you to pick up the pup as early as possible in the morning so that it will have all day to adjust to its new home. If you do not own a car, persuade a friend, preferably a close friend, into taking you. Should the whole family want to go with you, make sure there is room in the car for a deep cardboard box with an open top and some layers of old blankets, including an unwashed old sweater (if the 'chemistry' is right, the odour of the sweater will be a comfort to the pup). Instinctively, you will want to cradle this lonely, apprehensive little creature in your arms and, if you have children, they will be fighting over who is to hold the 'new puppy'. Desist! The puppy will probably throw up over you for a start, but there is a more important reason than preventing yourself smelling like a nasty hangover: by nursing the pup, you are immediately creating an overdependency. Many emotionally deprived people dote on their dogs and cannot stop cuddling and carrying them; consequently they spend half their lives tucked under their owners' arms so that you'd think they had been born with no legs! This is no good for owners or dogs.

The idea behind the cardboard box is that a box is easier to clean than you are but, more importantly, it emulates the 'cave' situation, making the pup feel secure. If the journey home is long, then take several short comfort stops. If the pup is carsick, which is often caused by stress rather than the motion of the car, play it cool but do *not* use a cooing, sympathetic voice to comfort the pup or it will become conditioned to turn on carsickness every time it travels.

Not only is travelling in itself a stressful experience but remember that the pup has just been engaged in strenuous litter play for the past two weeks. Leaving its litter mates and its mother and a situation where it had a definite position in the pack-order of the litter and some discipline from its dam is also a devastating experience for the pup. You and your family must bridge this gap as the pup's new replacement pack. The pup is very impressionable and easily confused at this stage as well as being totally dependent on you for food, water, shelter, leadership and emotional security. Now is the time to keep a delicate balance between allowing overdependency to develop and not providing enough emotional support.

Ideally, before the pup arrives home, there should be a family discussion in which tasks are delegated concerning the care of the pup, such as feeding, grooming, exercise and cleaning up the yard. Rostering the feeding to different members of the family means that the pup will learn to love you all and not become too dependent on any one person. If you do not have a family like one of those in an American soapie where the kids always end up listening to reason, you may experience some difficulty here, but persist! For people who live alone with their pup, the danger often is ending up with too much *mutual* dependency, so outside socialisation is important for both dog and owner.

## ARRIVING HOME

The first port of call on arriving home is the garden. The pup will probably relieve itself and if so, praise it. 'What a good dog,' in a cheery but not too over-the-top voice followed by a rub on the chest will do just fine. Patting a pup on the head is a dominant gesture in dog language and one that it will usually happily tolerate but a chest rub emulates mum rolling it over to give it a spit and polish after it has fed from her, so this gesture has much cosier associations.

If it is a dry day and the pup does not relieve itself, it may be persuaded to do so by pouring a little cold water on the ground and standing the pup's feet in it; with this 'puddle in order to piddle' technique, you are usually rewarded with the pup urinating. Again jolly but not overenthusiastic praise is in order.

It is now normal for the pup to investigate its surroundings and, as it does not know right from wrong, please remember it cannot be held morally responsible for its actions. If left unattended, it may dig, chew or be destructive to amuse itself. To avoid this, supervise the first play sessions. Say a firm 'No' and clap your hands to distract it from whatever it is doing that you consider to be wrong.

If isolated for long, the pup will whine to attract your attention. Obviously the pup must learn to adjust to spending time alone. A temporary pen is the way to help it do this. The pup will soon tire of exploring, so place it in a temporary pen with its first meal and some water in heavy broad-based containers that the pup can't knock over. Put the travelling cardboard box on its side, still with the layers of blanket and the unwashed sweater inside and, after putting the pup into the garden to relieve itself after its first meal, pop it back in the box inside the pen and go away.

By now rest will be needed and the pup will probably happily go to sleep. If it whines, this is perfectly normal behaviour as it is the pup's only form of communication to get your attention. It is still not acceptable behaviour however and, if allowed to go on, the pup may well turn into a barker as it matures. Emotional owners will reinforce this attention-getting behaviour by returning to placate and comfort the pup. Don't do it! A sharp rap on the side of the box is usually enough to stop it whining and also avoids the physical contact that the pup is seeking. This is not cruel. The temporary pen has good associations for the pup because it has been fed in it and now has a secure sleeping area, so it should settle in OK. The use of the pen can gradually be phased out as the pup grows into its new environment and way of life.

## SLEEPING ARRANGEMENTS: INSIDE OR OUT?

Many people start out by having their pup cosied up in the kitchen, taking precautions by having the floor spread with newspapers or else taking a resigned attitude to having the whole floor awash with wee in the morning. Apart from not being a good basis for house-training, this approach can have bad emotional repercussions for the pup. Owners often later ostracise the pup to outside accommodation when it gets bigger and this has disastrous results. Have you ever suffered rejection? It is as painful as grief and a dog feels it just as keenly. So start as you mean to continue. From the first night you must decide – is the pup to sleep inside or out?

Consider the case for keeping a dog inside the house. A dog is a pack animal. You have taken it away from this natural situation and therefore you have become its replacement pack. If a pup grows up in the house with you, for a start, there will be far fewer opportunities for it to indulge in such antics as archaeological excavations around your newly planted flower bed, swinging on your washing and constantly whining for attention. More importantly, such destructive and disturbed behaviour is a definite sign of separation anxiety. A pup will not suffer from this condition if it has company inside the house.

Consider also that your dog will be a far better burglar deterrent if it lives inside the house. Any experienced burglar knows if there is a dog locked in the backyard and he simply approaches from the other side of the house. Dogs who are perpetual barkers offer an excellent disguise to a break-in because the neighbours turn a deaf ear to a noisy dog who is always 'crying wolf', so to speak.

Let's dispel one myth, once and for all. A dog in a house is not a health hazard if regularly wormed. Loose dog-hair or a smelly dog can be a problem but the prevention of both these headaches is mainly a question of regular bathing and grooming for your dog.

Dogs have been companions to humans for centuries, gracing the hearths of feudal barons or the humbler households of more lowly folk. The dog is one of the few animals that has ever formed a really close relationship with human beings, so why miss out? As the chief object of owning a dog should be for companionship, it seems to defeat the whole point of the exercise to shut your dog out in the yard!

If this argument has not won you over, however, and you still insist on the dog sleeping outside, you will need to provide a good kennel. It should be insulated and raised from the ground so air can circulate underneath. Locate it by the back door. If not, the pup will probably set up camp by the back door anyway, regardless of wet or cold, to be near the last place that it saw you. Again, use your temporary pen as a small 'yard' in front of the kennel so the pup does not get into the habit of scratching on the back door when you are out. If the pup is to sleep in the kennel from its first night and you have put the pen in front of the kennel, then it will not be necessary to put the travelling cardboard box inside the kennel.

### Sleeping inside: a cosy solution

You have hopefully made the sensible decision to sleep your pup inside. For the first few nights, the travelling box should again be utilised. Put blankets in the bottom of the box and then place it on its side with the blanket hanging over the open side. For maximum effectiveness, the box should be placed totally upside down. Cut large ventilation holes in the sides but above the level where the pup can chew the cardboard edges of these holes. Then throw a blanket over the whole box to create such security that there won't be a peep out of the pup for hours. After about two nights, the box can then go on its side. After a few days, once the pup has settled in and feels secure, it may graduate to a basket.

Pups' bladders are like babies' bladders and, as you can't put a nappy

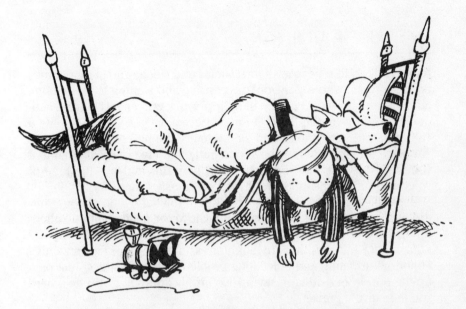

*Junior won't appreciate sharing his bed with the dog when it grows up.*

on a pup, it is worth having a night roster (about every four hours) to put the pup out. Mothers are usually up early in the morning and there is possibly a teenager home on the weekend, watching late-night movies, who can take care of the night shift, so you should all get enough sleep. As the pup grows, the bladder gains better control and bleary-eyed owners can get back to a normal cycle of sleep.

Some pups do unfortunately yell like banshees, even after you have done all the right things, including the old remedies of putting smelly sweaters, ticking clocks and hot-water bottles in the box, to no avail. Avoid at all costs Junior creeping downstairs and taking the pup to bed with him. Junior will later appreciate not having to share his bed with a huge Rottweiler when it grows up for he will be unwittingly training the pup to do just this later in life.

Put the upside-down box in your room but away from the bed as the bed can easily represent the 'den' or 'cave' of the dog family, which now means you and your family. In this way, the bed can become the scene of bitter power-games. A minute Maltese terrier got to the point of not letting the owner's politician husband come into bed with his wife after returning late from the House – by actually attacking him! Once the pup has settled in after a few nights, the box can be moved further away from the bedroom each night until the pup is sleeping where you first intended it to be, probably in the kitchen or laundry.

# HOUSE-TRAINING

A pup is likely to relieve itself after meals and sleeps and at other times usually gives a warning by looking pensive and starting to sniff about. Sometimes, however, it can be happily playing, wagging its tail and suddenly just do it on the floor. On most occasions you can anticipate a call of nature. After meals and sleeps, carry the pup outside to where you want it to go; you may have one particular area of the garden that you wish it to use. Praise the pup if it performs and use the tone of voice and rub on the chest described previously (page 76).

If it makes a mistake and you catch it in the act, on no account rub the pup's nose in the urine or slap it, however gently, with a rolled-up newspaper. This sort of approach went out with the Ark. Corporal punishment and shouting are highly stressful to dogs and in fact cause abnormal urinating and defecating problems through stress. Just pick up the pup in mid-stream, saying 'No' firmly and put it outside where you then give it praise.

'So you think I can do this all day and that I've nothing better to do with my time?' a harassed Mrs Henderson said to me when she brought her 7-week-old new pup to the surgery for its first shots.

'Not at all,' I replied, 'but let some domestic chores slide for a few days. You can have one eye on the pup and one eye on the cheese grater and surely no one will notice if there's a bit of your finger in the cheese soufflé! It really pays to work hard for just a few days with great consistency, especially as you have a family that can take it in turns. It will save your pup from developing bad behaviour patterns, prevent carpets being stained, and will avoid a problem that may never be solved later on. It is just a question of building up a conditioned reflex in your dog.'

Mrs Henderson went away muttering, 'It's all very well for that vet. I wonder what sort of mess her house is in!'

What if you haven't a yard? And what do you do when it is pouring with rain outside? You know that old song that goes 'and her bathing suit never got wet'? Well, that describes some dogs for you. Even when house-trained, they take one look at the wet weather, emit a deep sigh and you see their abdomen swell visibly as the wet day progresses; others think, 'To hell with it! I'm not going out in that rain. I'll sneak upstairs' and they go off to find some secret corner for their business.

To train pups who live in flats or who are trapped inside on rainy days, newspaper is the answer. Dogs are attracted to the chemical smell in newspaper print and can be happily placed on the paper at the appropriate times and then duly praised.

Now there are a few traps here. Take the case of one of my clients who was a psychiatrist and should have known better. The family had paper-trained their dog and there was the owner enjoying his Sunday morning croissant and coffee, with the weekend tabloids strewn all over the floor around his chair. In came Adler and promptly deposited a turd on the Stock Market Report. The owner went berserk but then, he had trained his dog to do just that, hadn't he? The same rule applies if you are taking your dog for a walk and it is not leashed and you pass a newsagency with a pile of virgin newspapers hurled on the pavement. Your dog's eyes light up and off he charges to christen the bunch of newspapers. Anticipate this potentially embarrassing episode by sidling past the newsagency with your dog firmly on a leash.

## PLAYTIME

Plain boredom is a problem with dogs, so toys are appreciated to keep them amused. Choose carefully however. There are currently on the market nylon, scented bones that, unlike beef-hide ones, are virtually indestructible. They have an odour that is attractive to the puppy so it will continually go back and chew the bone, thus helping to relieve boredom and also provide an outlet for the pup's increased desire to chew as its gums get sore from teething. However a minority of pups do not take to these bones.

Be very wary of what other toys you give the pup to play with. The owner of a Great Dane rang me, sounding quite hysterical, 'Hamlet has got hold of a pair of very expensive imported Italian shoes and he is demolishing them right in front of me. I tried to get them off him but he went for me!' Now, you could not really blame Hamlet for eating those shoes. He had been given a whole range of old shoes to play with as a puppy, so to him all shoes were fair game.

All rubber toys and old things are out of the question because pups can chew them up and swallow them. A small rubber ball, the size of a golf ball, almost caused the demise of a German shepherd dog I treated; it got stuck hard at the entrance to his windpipe. On arrival at the surgery he was purple-tongued and in a state of collapse. Thankfully, we managed to dislodge it and save the dog from suffocation.

There is on the market a tug-of-war game which, in our professional view, should be banned. It encourages pups to seize and hold with devastating results. Children, especially boys, and men (many of whom are just big kids, anyway) love to rough play with pups, grabbing them by the mouth and shaking them from side to side. It may seem amusing to see this tiny roly-poly pup growling like an adult dog in mock play and you think you have a 'real character' on your hands but these mouth and tug-of-war games turn out to be deadly serious if allowed to go on. At sexual maturity, and often before, this learned and encouraged behaviour will turn to biting. If the pup tries to chew at your hands, do not snatch them away but remove them slowly out of sight behind your back. This will calmly but firmly discourage 'biting' games.

Another game with dangerous consequences is playing chasings. Children love this game: the pup madly dashes after them and they all end up in a tumbled tangle on the ground. Delightful though this child–pup rapport may seem, it can end up one day with a complaint to the police that a dog chased and bit someone's child. The poor dog, in such a case, is simply obeying his natural chase-and-catch instinct that has been unwittingly overencouraged by its owners from an early age.

'But my children will be so bored. They won't be able to play naturally with the pup,' you may say. They can still have fun in more constructive ways. They can throw objects for the pup to retrieve and take it for walks on a lead. And what about those marvellous moments of togetherness when children cuddle up in front of the telly with a sleeping pup? We need to remember that with a dominant dog it is unwise to be on the same level with it. To be above means to be dominant for this type of dog.

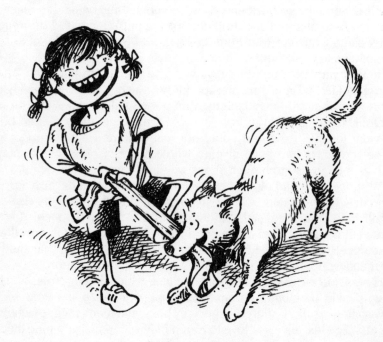

*Don't encourage this!*

If you start by nursing a pup on your lap and later it grows too big, it will feel rejected. I was a victim of this mistake. I gave a home to an adult 40-kilogram Weimaraner. He kept climbing on my lap and winding himself round my neck during thunderstorms. The walls could have fallen down around me but, with my circulation at a standstill, I was completely immobilised. Sure enough, I found out from the previous owner that he had been nursed on her lap as a puppy. Luckily for me, as he became more secure, this annoying behaviour ceased.

## REST: FOR DOG AND OWNER

Pups will play madly and then get restless and whinge like an overtired toddler and need putting to bed. With a human infant, you hear mothers say, 'I'm just going to put baby down now.' This sort of expression produces some startled looks from vets who are used to hearing their clients say, 'Does my dog have to be put down?', meaning of course euthanasia!

Even the prestigious London department store, Harrods, closes its doors in the puppy sales department twice a day so that the pups get proper rest. It has been shown that without a stable environment the development of nervous tissue, organ size and the chemical balance of a dog's body can all be affected, setting the scene for poor health and the beginnings of delinquent behaviour.

If you have children who wake up a pup to play whenever the mood takes them or when they come home from school, you will have an overstimulated and exhausted pup who will grow up into a hyperactive dog. This can be as bad as living with a hyperactive child. It's almost worse in fact, as you don't get a reprieve as you do when a child is away at school all day plus, if the dog's big enough, you get knocked over all the time as well!

## LONELINESS: PARTING IS SUCH SWEET SORROW

One of the most common mistakes people make is to take time off work to devote to a new puppy in order to settle it in. Even just one whole weekend of overindulging a pup with attention can result in 'Monday madness' when the fretful pup, once left alone, will proceed to tear up everything in sight and scream its head off.

So to start, put the pup in its temporary pen and then all of you go about your own business away from the pup. It will soon learn to feel secure when alone for reasonable periods and not indulge in so-called separation anxiety behaviour. From the first day, all go out, even just for a little while. A pup soon learns to identify the actions of its owners. Some dogs, when they see the owner shutting up the windows, collecting their belongings and generally getting ready to go out, plant themselves by the front door with an anxious look in an endeavour not to be left behind.

Many owners increase the dog's stress in this situation by indulging in an almost tearful guilty farewell before they go. This sort of farewell will seem to the pup as something that it should feel really bad about, so of course it does. The resultant howls bring the owner back for further comforting, only to exacerbate the situation even more.

A dog's uncanny powers of observation and excellent memory teach it many things. A dog who loves going in the car will react with joy at the rattle of the car keys in the same way that the sound of its food dishes will bring it running for a meal. By learning your habits of dress and behaviour, a pup grows up to know if it is to accompany you on an outing or not. If I get dressed up to go out in 'non-dog walk' clothes, my dog just emits a deep sigh and drops down disgustedly with an 'I'm-going-to-slit-my-wrists' look. One client's dog gets wildly excited when she goes towards the door at a certain time because he knows that he is being taken out but at other times he will not react at all because she has a shopping bag in her hand.

There was one particlar dog who was becoming a 'problem child' whenever the owner went out. He was perfectly happy however when he saw her leave with a pile of dirty washing under her arm because he knew she would only be gone for half an hour or so down in the laundry in the block of flats. Because he thus associated dirty washing with her returning in a short while, his destructive sessions in her absence were easily cured. Now, whenever she goes to the shops or further afield, she always leaves carrying some dirty washing under her arm, then dumps it outside until her return. The happily deluded dog no longer tears the place apart!

Get a regular routine established if you are going to work every day and leaving the dog. Give it its morning meal, have a play, clean up the yard, change the water and then clean up once more after its breakfast before you leave.

Many pups get into the habit of eating their own droppings. This is utterly repulsive in human terms but perfectly normal for some pups. They have observed their mother eat the litter's droppings, which is survival behaviour to conceal the pups' presence from predators and, imitating mum, they can grow to like the taste of it if it becomes a habit. When the faeces have been on the ground for a while they hatch worm eggs that become infective, so a dog eating its droppings (or those of other dogs) is in danger of infection. The habit of coprophagia (as eating droppings is called) is one that the pup usually outgrows, but it is best never to create the opportunity for it to indulge in the habit. If this behaviour persists in older dogs, along with such habits as eating rubbish and licking concrete, the dog may have a genuine mineral deficiency, worms or else a lack of certain digestive enzymes. This is a case for the vet. Coprophagia is also an outlet for stress in dogs.

# A GOOD RELATIONSHIP: THE PERFECT OWNER

Pups, just like children, are opportunists and they will quickly pick up on an inconsistent owner and take advantage of the situation. They can also suffer as a result. Pups are very sensitive to mood swings of owners and this can often build insecurity in the pup, which then indulges in stress-relieving activities such as digging and chewing. In severe cases, stress can lead to self-mutilation such as tail-chasing and chewing, the constant licking of paws and tail and the chewing of the front leg, which can produce a potentially malignant ulcer.

Inconsistent moods and behaviour patterns in an owner lead to a breakdown in a dog's respect for pack-leadership; equally, an indifferent attitude from the owner can produce the same response from the pup. This loss of respect leads to the owner's frustration with his or her pet, which in turn builds up more stress in the pup resulting in further problem behaviour.

Dogs whose owners hit the bottle often become emotionally disturbed wrecks. One woman was always happy and cheerful after a few drinks and let her children and pup do whatever they liked. But the next morning, when the euphoria had worn off and the hangover had set in, the pup got bawled at as well as the kids – for no apparently good reason. A pup goes through a fear imprint stage between the age of 8 and 10 weeks and a traumatic experience to a stressed puppy at this time can affect its behaviour for the rest of its adult life.

One day a little old man, who lived in a boarding house, came to see me with his Yorkshire terrier. I could not at first understand why he got so worked up when I went to wipe the surgery table with disinfectant, a routine between all cases. 'Don't put any alcohol on it. It makes him go mad!' I unscrambled the mystery: the caretaker of the boarding house was an alcoholic and every time the little old man came into the building the caretaker would abuse and scream at the dog who would, if not restrained, try to bite his attacker. This was a fear response on behalf of the dog, imprinted from an early age because of the aggressive behaviour of the drunk. It was not the smell of liquor alone that was sending the dog completely off its head but the associated trauma!

If your pup is doing something unreasonable, do not get mad at it but look for the reason in doggy terms. This will give you an opportunity to keep calm and deal with the problem correctly. Many so-called 'cures' for bad dog behaviour, such as putting the dog's droppings in the hole he has dug in the garden, have been written about but most of these can cause nasty side effects without in fact curing the original behaviour problem. The patience that results from attempting to understand a dog's point of view will ultimately build a more stable relationship between dog and owner. Of course if we could all be compassionate, understanding, tolerant, emotionally stable dog owners, some of these attributes might rub off on our human relationships!

5

# Nutrition and Diet

## CANINE CUISINE: WHAT AND HOW MUCH?

It was a familiar voice on the phone – Mrs Carlson, whose previous dog had finally been put down with terminal cancer when he was 16 years old. Many people feel they are being disloyal to the memory of their old dog if they get another one, but the Carlsons realised that the natural life span of a dog is far less than ours so it is quite natural for us to own several in our lifetime. Something had to fill the empty gap and the good memories of Zola would not be diminished. Sensibly, there were no unfair expectations of the new pup by comparing it with Zola. Life with the new dog was to be treated as a clean slate.

'We only got her from the kennels yesterday!' said Mrs Carlson. 'She has had her first shots but I am thoroughly thrown by the diet sheet the breeder has given me. Why, I'd need to retire from work to have the time just to prepare it! What do *you* think I should feed her?'

I'd seen many a sample of breeders' diets before and wondered how they could claim to be professionals when the results were too often unhealthy pups with poor bone. Some ingredients in breeders' sheets have merit such as garlic, which is good for the body's defence system and contains oils that help get rid of worms. But who has the time to stand at a kitchen bench with a garlic crusher preparing ingredients for a dog meat loaf or stew? Most reputable breeders, however, feed good-quality canned food mixed with dried food that is nutritionally balanced.

I told Mrs Carlson to feed the new pup about three or four small meals a day, two canned and two complete dried food, and to leave fresh water available at all times. Pups decide for themselves the number of meals per day that they require just as human infants do. But when it comes to each particular meal, a pup's eyes are usually bigger than its tummy, so never let it eat as much as it wants. Quantities on cans and packets are a rough guide but each individual pup has different needs, in the same way that some people have a voracious appetite and never get fat while others *look* at a doughnut and begin to spread. Experiment with quantities so that the pup is not overdistended in the abdomen or groaning after a meal. A dog should not be pot-bellied nor have its ribs showing. A trim, healthy physique is ideal.

Don't worry if a pup gets an attack of hiccoughs after dinner. Hiccoughs can be quite normal in pups and are caused by intermittent contractions of the diaphragm. If they persist however the cause could be worms. Pups with worms may bolt their food very fast because they are perpetually hungry; their worms have cashed in on the free meal ticket.

# IT'S IN THE CAN:
# A FEW QUESTIONS ANSWERED

International pet-food companies of good standing have spent vast sums of money in research on nutrition. Veterinary schools throughout the world and the National Research Council have confirmed that the feeding of good-quality commercial canned food is properly balanced and adequate nutritionally for the majority of dogs. In this day and age, few people have the time to do much more than wield the can-opener for their pets. There are some questions, however, about canned food that should be answered.

*Don't cans contain substances detrimental to health and lacking in vitamins?*
The manufacturers of many commercial foods have cut out all colouring matter and preservatives in their products that can be responsible for some skin allergies later in a dog's life. Colouring matter in dog food is often only caramel and not synthesised chemicals. Most cans of better-quality pet food add extra vitamins to make up for any vitamin loss during the sterilisation process.

Occasionally there are some dogs whose immune systems become deficient as they get older, so then there is some justification for switching to raw whole foods but these cases are the exception to the rule. On the whole, canned food is adequate. We commonly make the mistake of comparing canned human food to canned pet food. No one would dream of feeding their child on canned food alone, so some owners believe the same should go for their other 'child', the family dog. But pet food is in fact far more nutritious than most canned human food so that we end up with the grim result that pets in affluent countries are better fed than most children!

*But isn't a diet of canned and dried food too boring?*
The short answer is no. A human baby's taste buds are very sensitive; a little salt makes them screw up their tiny faces. Pups also have highly sensitive palates – which never forget! If you start a pup on non-commercial food, it will refuse to ever go back to the commercial stuff, behaving as if it had been offered a plate of poison! Start a dog's diet as you mean to continue.

Unless encouraged to eat fine foods when young, dogs are not, however, naturally fussy eaters. *You* might get bored (among other things) with baked beans on toast every day of the week but a dog will happily eat the same thing all the time if it has not been spoilt with sophisticated gastronomical delights as are some French pooches. An art-deco restaurant in Nice, which catered exclusively for dogs, served its doggy guests diced turkey, creme caramel and a range of cheeses. Apparently the canine 'patrons' were not impressed with the venue, probably due to the threateningly close proximity of their fellow diners.

Puppies double their weight very quickly, particularly the larger breeds, so they will eat twice the amount that a fully grown dog does on a comparable weight basis. For this reason there are special cans formulated for puppies only that contain far higher quantities of meat than do cans for adult dogs so that puppies receive adequate protein for optimum growth. The correct amount of calcium has been added to make up for its deficiency in meat, together with the correct quantities of fat, carbohydrate, protein and minerals. These cans are also useful for dogs in convalescence or old age.

*Is a diet only of canned food enough?*
Tiny erupting teeth need something to chew on. There are high-protein, balanced, complete dry foods for puppies on the market that are not quite as hard as the dried food for adult dogs. Be advised by your vet about the best brand as most non-generic brands are not adequate nutritionally.

*Is what's on the can in the can?*
When you look at the ingredients printed on the label of a can of dog food, you will notice most brands contain approximately the same percentages of the different ingredients, regardless of price. It is the

*quality* of these ingredients that is not stated. A rough guide to quality is to poke about in the contents and see what you can see! Arteries like drain-pipes, lumps of gritty bone, a lot of sloshy background without much solids, or bits of skin, mean that the available protein is low as the meat is obviously of poor quality. If a dog passes bulky stools on a new diet or breaks wind even after he has got used to the change to a new diet, this may indicate poor-quality meat also. Most cans have about 7 per cent protein on a wet basis which, with the rest of the solids, adds up to about 10 per cent solids. You are buying an awful lot of water with every can of pet food!

Also, be aware that the amount of protein is often estimated on the nitrogen content, which is also present in hoof and horn. It does not take much brain power to work out that this sort of mix is not as body-building as a hunk of steak. As a result, the percentage of crude proteins listed on the label may be deceptive.

Any large pet-food company that has extensive research laboratories will produce a good product. Often there are so-called gourmet brands. They touch the heart of the owner who buys them with an anticipatory glow of pleasure at the delight it will give their dog. The ingredients in these products do not comprise a complete diet, but they certainly have a captive market.

### Hand-feeding: once bitten, twice shy
Should you have a pup who is nervous or has been sick and you think needs coaxing with food, never make the mistake of hand-feeding it. Your pup will eat when it is good and ready. Hand-fed puppies will have to be hand-fed all their lives. Of course, some owners love this dependency as it makes them feel wanted.

### Why not a natural diet?
What is a dog's natural diet? The wild ancestral dog would catch prey, tear open the abdomen and probably first eat the offal such as the liver, rich in vitamins A, D, B and iron. It then ate the intestines that contained, in the case of a herbivorous animal like a rabbit, vegetables already partly digested. Then it would devour the muscles and bones, demolishing the skin as well, which probably afforded some protection against splinters of bone. Wolves in the wild eat berries off trees. This curious fact makes it easier to understand why a colleague's dachshund used to stuff itself with mulberries fallen from their mulberry bush and then pass some alarmingly coloured stools!

But a person's idea of feeding a natural diet for a dog usually means meat and vegetables. Meat alone is very low in calcium and this can result in a flat-footed, hump-backed and 'cow-hocked' adult dog. Raw vegetables often irritate the gut and cause diarrhoea. A swallowed corn cob for example cannot be digested by the dog and may have to be surgically removed.

*I still won't feed my dog canned food!*
It is sometimes hard to break the prejudice against commercially prepared food. Many people would never dream of opening a can for themselves so they won't for their dog. People can't help judging the nutritional value of canned pet food from their viewpoint of canned food for human consumption. There is, as I said before, no comparison because good-quality pet food has been scientifically balanced to make a complete diet.

If you are still not convinced, however, you can feed raw meat (not offal) with a teaspoon of calcium carbonate per 125 grams weight. Add a little maize oil or lard and a sprinkling of brewer's yeast. This diet can be supplemented with cottage cheese and the occasional hard-boiled egg. Additional vegetables should be cooked, not raw.

# DIET: ALTERNATIVES AND ADDITIONS

*I'm a vegetarian; can my dog be too?*
A dog is a natural carnivore. It has large canine, or fang, teeth for seizing and tearing prey, huge molars for grinding and tiny front incisors because . . . well, they are of little use! A dog isn't a horse or cow, who needs massive incisors to crop grass. Although canned foods appear to be unnatural, the ingredients have been properly balanced to give the correct formula for a carnivorous diet. Most vegetarians can justify opening a can of meat on the grounds that they are feeding a natural carnivore while avoiding the aesthetic problem of having to cut up raw meat themselves. Admittedly this is something of an 'ostrich-with-its-head-in-the-sand' attitude, similar to that held by most people who prefer not to think of the small lamb, gambolling in the springtime field with its playmates, when they sit down to eat lamb chops. For those vegetarians more deeply troubled by their consciences, it is possible to have a healthy vegetarian dog but not a vegan dog, that is to say, a dog on a diet without dairy products or eggs. The Vegetarian Society of Great Britain publishes a pamphlet that gives diets for vegetarian dogs and cats.

Dogs seem to thrive on a morning meal of wholegrain cereal and milk and an evening meal of high-protein foods such as ground nuts, cheese, legumes or textured vegetable protein mixed with raw or cooked vegetables. Variation can be supplied with brown rice, whole-wheat bread, sprouts, fruit, wholegrain biscuits or raw, whole carrots for the dog's teeth.

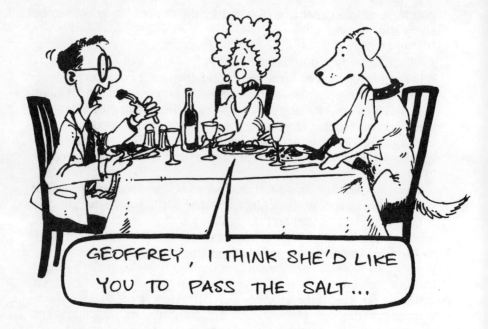

GEOFFREY, I THINK SHE'D LIKE YOU TO PASS THE SALT...

### 'She only eats what we eat': international cuisine

Dogs belonging to Asian families are quite happily adjusted to curries while Italian pooches slurp down spaghetti. They are used to it so their digestive systems have learned to cope. Sudden changes to food with spices, wine and herbs, however, can cause diarrhoea.

Some table scraps are fine as long as they are fresh and your dog won't even mind a dollop of custard on the stew! Do not feed human leftovers until after 9 months of age as a balanced diet of good commercially prepared pet food is the best start in life for proper physical development. Once a pup has tasted the gastronomical novelty and richness of human foods, it may resort to blackmail and refuse to ever eat commercial pet foods again. So you have been warned! A dog's health can be in danger if over 20 per cent of its diet consists of table scraps.

### Titbits: not a good idea

Mrs Jenkins lived alone with her pug. He was portly even for a pug (and they are a terribly gluttonous breed). Mrs Jenkins had a weight problem. She had arthritis, which did not encourage her to walk enough with her dog, so they both got bored and sublimated their boredom with food. There was toast and vegemite for breakfast. Then morning tea with lamingtons and a hot dog at lunchtime; a sticky bun at afternoon tea, meat and two veg. at dinnertime and biscuits with a saucer of cocoa at bedtime. A dog in the wild will catch prey, gorge himself and then not eat anything for a couple of days. No wonder Chin Chin suffered from wind and had no waistline! When I tackled Mrs Jenkins on the subject of the excessive number of titbits, her face fell visibly.

'But I couldn't eat in front of him! Why I'd hardly eat at all!' she wailed. That might not be at all a bad idea I thought but held my tongue. This togetherness over the food ritual was so important to Mrs Jenkins that I decided to let the issue go but begged her to cut down Chin Chin's own meals by half. This way they could continue their gastronomical trysts but with smaller amounts, comprising not more than 20 per cent of Chin Chin's diet. If she hadn't cut his weight down, then every morsel would have been another coffin nail for this unhealthy pug.

From the first day that you get a new pup home, never be tempted to feed titbits from the table. If you do, the dog will pester you at every meal. It will learn to fix you with a melting look and imploringly paw you with its foot, a cleverly disguised dominant gesture from a dog. If you live alone, like Mrs Jenkins, and you really must feed titbits, then go ahead. For a family or for any person who entertains guests, however, you will find that your visitors will not appreciate your dog's undivided attention at the dinner table.

The elderly are particularly prone to overindulging their dogs and sometimes at the expense of their own health and diet. Miss Larkin was elderly, existing on only a tiny pension, but she gave her Pomeranian, Lucy, the best-quality grilling steak. I looked at her bony wrists and her paper-thin skin and thought to myself, 'You need that good-quality food because Lucy will do just as well on cheaper cuts, with calcium added of course.' Many elderly people go without food for the sake of their pets for the totally wrong reasons. Miss Larkin even cut every bit of fat off her Pom's steak, thinking she was doing the right thing, when in fact some fat in a dog's diet is necessary to transport the fat-soluble vitamins in the body.

### Stealing food: also a bad idea

The simple rule about stealing food is to never give a pup the opportunity to do so. After many years I thought I could trust my dog. Then one day he ate a whole pâté that I had slaved over simply because I'd left it on a low coffee table, in preparation for my guests, while I was in the kitchen. When he'd finished wolfing it down, the bowl didn't look as if it even needed washing! Keep food out of temptation's way.

### Oversupplementing with minerals and vitamins

Human health freaks fill their puppies with vitamins and mineral supplements, often with disastrous results. Excess vitamin D in a dog's diet can cause bone deformity. Overfeeding a dog calcium can cause deposits of unwanted calcium in all the wrong places. Excess iron can cause bowel damage and loss of weight. Breeders of large dogs often oversupplement with minerals with exactly the opposite result from that which they had hoped to achieve, namely deformed bones instead of sound ones. A balanced diet does not need supplementing. Also, excessive food consumption can accelerate growth rate and thereby enhance the development of the inherited condition of hip dysplasia.

### No bones about it

Certainly, dogs can have fun with bones. Chewing and grinding them up fulfils natural instincts for bone-crunching and also can be a great reliever of boredom for the urban dog. The wild dog may grind up rabbits, rodents and birds without coming to any harm because such dogs are conditioned to it but our city-slicker dogs are somewhat softer and certain bones can cause a lot of problems, especially in the very young. Chops and T-bones can get stuck, while passing down the oesophagus (or gullet) on their way to the stomach, at three main junctions: at the entrance to the chest; inside the thoracic cavity near the heart; or at the diaphragm. Bones cannot get digested in the oesophagus so they have to be surgically removed. Rabbit bones can be dangerous and chicken bones splinter. All bones for dogs to chew on should be large, such as lamb shanks, and they should be fed raw. Dogs under a year old shouldn't be left alone with a bone as they are inexperienced and can easily get into trouble. Hunks of bone can get jammed on the molars and rib-bones can get stuck across the roof of the mouth where the jaw narrows.

### Some big taboos

Don't feed puppies human baby food. Don't feed them kangaroo meat, not only on conservation grounds, but because it hasn't been properly inspected and often carries salmonella infection. It also does not contain enough fat for a dog's diet. Some pups cannot digest cow's milk as they may lack the enzyme lactase to digest the milk-sugar lactose and this causes diarrhoea. Although mainly occurring in older dogs, some foods may cause allergies. These include milk, beef, wheat products and semi-soft packaged pet food. Because of the semi-soft consistency of the latter, preservatives have been included and these can cause a skin allergy in some dogs.

Food is fantastic, most of us would agree. Gourmet delights tempt many of us and the human condition is such that we may overindulge as an outlet for our emotions. Dogs will too and many reflect the eating habits of their owners. It is your choice if you want to make a rod for your own back by indulging your dog or whether you want to feed it a sensible diet designed for the canine palate. Remember, your dog will not miss what it hasn't had – and it cannot read epicurean cookbooks!

# 6

# How to Survive the First Four Months

## PATIENCE IS A PREREQUISITE

Do you yell at the kids to stop watching telly but then let them go on watching anyway? Do you walk out on the boss in a bad mood, slamming the door behind you? Are you a teenager who throws things in a tantrum? Or are you an elderly person with the habit of worrying about everything, even minor problems? If so, your potential for raising a well-adjusted pup is just about nil! This is because an owner's inconsistency, unpredictable swinging moods and lack of constant leadership will result in an insecure pup. The pup then suffers from stress, which is expressed in the form of destructive behaviour such as digging, chewing, yapping and barking.

It is rarely possible to change a person's basic personality but if you are aware that you are someone who has a short fuse, you can modify your reactions to a pup's annoying behaviour simply by trying to understand why your pup has behaved as it has on its own terms. In this way, you will regain control and the pup's respect. Admittedly, this is not easy when you come home after a tough day and find feathers from a chewed pillow floating through the room like a gentle fall of snow. Acknowledge it was your fault for leaving the pillow in the path of temptation and take a deep breath!

# THE MIND OF A 6-WEEK-OLD PUP

A pup cannot talk or reason and possesses no moral standards in human terms. You have become the replacement for its mother who gave it constant direction and taught it to understand the rules of the litter. If pup stepped out of line, mother would correct it. This doesn't mean you have to pick up the pup by the scruff of the neck in your mouth and give it a shake. A simple 'No' in a low tone will do the trick.

You must not only watch your own reactions to a pup's behaviour but, if you have children, you have to keep an eye on them as well. Too often an animal is the brunt of someone else's redirected ill humour. Little Simon had been given a slap on the behind by his father because he tipped his cereal on his head. He ran from the room, yelling his head off, and promptly hit the family's inoffensive puppy. This sort of behaviour can cause great psychological damage to a pup and should be watched for and strictly discouraged.

Pups are smart. A tiny pup can be very knowing and, like a young baby, quickly learns to stop crying when it is picked up. It is cunning enough to manipulate you emotionally and become a four-legged leader in a two-legged pack. Your puppy also has incredible powers of observation. It will read your body language with deadly accuracy, which is

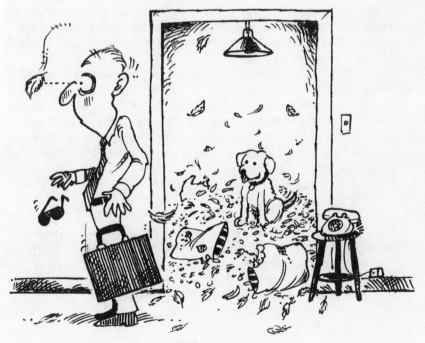

*Keep your cool.*

more than can be said for most owners, who do not understand their dog's body language at all.

The pup will observe situations and react accordingly. For example, it will become animated when you open the fridge door because it anticipates food. This can give you a false idea of the pup's present ability to be trained because it is really only displaying a specific reaction to a self-learned situation. *You* can take no credit for directing such stimulus–response behaviour.

## TRAINING A 6-WEEK-OLD PUP

Mrs Walker complained that their pup did not seem to get the message when her family told it not to do something. No wonder! Mr Walker would say, 'Stop that at once, sir!' in true British public-school tradition. Mrs Walker herself yelled, 'Cut that out!' while their daughter cooed, 'Oh, you naughty little darling' in a voice that clearly indicated that it was fine by her. Not surprisingly, the pup became totally confused and pursued its destructive games with renewed vigour without understanding that they were a 'no-no'. And that is the operative word – a 'No' spoken in a low tone.

Sometimes, but only very occasionally, a louder voice may be effective as a restraining influence when the fun of what the pup has been up to has made it temporarily deaf! Using a constantly loud voice to correct a dog becomes completely ineffectual as you have nothing left to fall back on for a sterner reproach.

Making the pup do something positive, as opposed to *stopping* it doing something, usually has to be carried out with a physical action by you such as putting the pup in its basket and at the same time saying 'basket'. The pup gets to know the sound of the word by association. If you are consistent in this approach, your dog when it is older will go straight to its basket when you say the word, albeit sometimes with a resigned sigh.

With constant repetition, your pup will get to know many key words. It is vitally important to know, however, that a pup under the age of 4 months cannot retain any training. It would be rather like expecting a 2-year-old child to bring you the postman's delivery mail every day without fail! Because a pup appears to have forgotten what it has been taught, the owner sometimes gets angry and frustrated. The sight of a cross owner, looming tall and menacing, can be very threatening to a pup. Please have patience and realistic expectations.

## TAKING THE LEAD

Although formal obedience training should not be started until the pup is at least 16 weeks old, it should be introduced to the lead from about 6 weeks of age. A light leather or webbing lead should be attached to a collar of similar material. Some pups walk on the lead immediately. Others perform handstands and cartwheels, tangle up themselves and you, roll on their backs, grab the lead and try to chew through it and dig in their heels and refuse to move, as if you were trying to drag them over a precipice. In this case attach the lead and let the pup drag it around under supervision just to get used to the fact that it is not an enemy.

When your pup is so young, do not use either a chain-lead or a choke-chain. These types of lead are noisy and frighten some pups and, if the pup attacks a chain-lead, it can knock out delicately erupting teeth; the resulting pain will create an aversion to all leads, never to be forgotten.

It is worthwhile to take a little time to break in to lead work and, once a good association with the lead has been built up, the pup will look forward to its walks. Wait until about ten days after the pup's first vaccination shots before taking it into the outside world. Remember, however, that this vaccine may not be protecting it very strongly so discourage the pup from sniffing around lamp posts and trees where there is a concentration of urine and faeces that could carry disease. Sometimes on the first walk it is best to carry the pup a short way and then let it be led back home.

## THE BIG BAD WORLD OUTSIDE

Many a pup, born with a good temperament and with no problems interacting with other pups in its litter, can still grow up as a nervous adult because of lack of experience outside its backyard environment. It is illegal in most, if not all, parts of the world to let dogs out alone. They are therefore dependent on you to give them walks for exercise and to expose them to interaction with the outside environment. This exposure plays a vital part in shaping a dog's character.

If something frightens the wits out of a pup between 8 and 10 weeks of age, it may scare the dog for the rest of its life. This is called fear imprinting. When a pup walks down the road for the first time, it will come across all sorts of experiences that we take for granted: children running and laughing, skateboards, bikes, car doors slamming, flapping garbage bags, gratings, open stairways, bridges, sounds of the wind, hollow sounds of footsteps, the hot air currents and noise when a bus races past. These are all strange and potentially scary sights and sounds.

Wobbly things to walk on worry pups too, and not only pups. I had a 10-year-old German shepherd dog who suddenly froze and dropped trembling when I walked her on a wooden ramp around a swimming pool. The sight of the water between the planks frightened her. Then one day I took some foxhounds into a television studio for a dog programme and they refused to move in the lino corridors. You can feel pretty silly carrying a foxhound! Stone walls and rivers might be taken quite happily in their stride but not slippery floors!

Jim once trained a pup for a woman who wanted to walk it beside her baby's stroller. The dog's reluctance to do so was soon fixed by oiling the wheels of the stroller. Although it was not obvious to the owner, the pup's more acute hearing, made even more sensitive by being low to the ground, amplified the squeaking of the stroller's wheels to an unbearable pitch. An owner must be sensitive to all the forbidding sights and sounds of the outside world from a young pup's point of view.

So, your pup on its first outings is under constant threat and, of course, you cannot explain to it that there is nothing to be scared of. If you yourself were in a frightening situation, you would be much happier if you were with a person who took charge of the situation with confidence than with someone who was as worried as you were. Such anxiety does not create good leadership and confident leadership is exactly what the pup needs. So don't worry about the pup being worried but instead jolly it up and proceed in a calm manner. Soon the pup will gain confidence too and will begin to accept all sorts of situations without reacting. If you use a soothing, sympathetic voice, however, you will just reinforce its fear.

I remember once seeing a cocker spaniel pup happily chewing its carry basket in the Paris metro amidst the thunderous noise. Then, at the next stop, a rather nervous man got in the carriage, carrying a large German shepherd pup that was shaking like a jelly. I thought how he is going to love carrying that dog when it's fully grown because, if he does not change his attitude now, that is precisely what he will be doing in a few years time!

Many irresponsible owners let their dogs roam and such dogs may become very territorial in their own street and will challenge you in an aggressive way as you pass their property while out on a walk with your pup. This could well upset your pup but it is most unlikely that the older dog will do much more than inspect your pup with a sniff; your pup is quite neutral sexually at this early age and poses no threat to older dogs. Once you realise this fact, you can reassure the pup and walk firmly on. As you both leave the other dog's territory, it will immediately lose interest. Your pup may behave in a scared or submissive manner, even rolling on its back, but try not to pick it up. Just wait and encourage it to walk on.

# RECALL WORK

Recall work should be started at a very early age and in a park. Walk away from the pup, calling to it encouragingly and then praising it when it reaches you. As the pup is highly dependent on you when it is very young, you can condition it to come quickly on demand from a very early age. The small creature's dependency makes you feel really good! You are making the most of the leadership potential that you will need to firmly bring the dog into line when it gets older. If you wait until it is older, however, before attempting any sort of restraint training, the pup will have developed no respect for you and will show this clearly by becoming aggressive if crossed.

Many young pup-owners, who may live in just one room, will usually take the pup everywhere with them. I often see a tiny pup limping along behind such owners, desperately trying to keep up with them while off the leash, frequently on a crowded city street. If a tiny pup receives exercise at this level, its bones, which are growing and still not hard and calcified, will become very sore and the pup will become lame. Short but frequent walks is the only way to exercise a pup, even right up to one year of age.

When a small pup or even an adult dog does what it has been told, you, the owner, are usually so overcome and delighted that you over-react with lavish praise and say things like 'Oh, what a good dog, aren't you a clever dog?' and so on. This acts as a release from any discipline and the pup goes absolutely crazy with joy and jumps all over you, covering you with wet kisses. Just hand out brief low-key praise. A quick rub around the ear and a murmured 'good boy' is adequate reward. This way, the dog keeps its mind on the job and does not lose its concentration during the critical training period.

# CHAOS WHILE YOU'RE OUT: PREVENTION

Curiosity and the need for a thorough investigation of its surroundings are high on a pup's list of priorities. This urge to explore can create such havoc that if you leave a large pup on the loose in an out-of-bounds space when you go out, the resultant mayhem will stun you when you get home. It is natural to feel and express anger at this point, but this is totally self-defeating. What the puppy has done is, for better or worse, perfectly normal behaviour in a pup.

The solution is to create a 'safe' area where there are no plants, garden furniture, poisonous garden preparations, or anything that you do not want damaged. If you have a garden that doesn't have aspirations to be in *Vogue* magazine, then just wire off the areas that are forbidden, particularly where you have planted new shrubs because newly turned soil immediately attracts pups with all the new smells that have been exposed. If you are in fact a *House and Garden* aspirant, then wire in a small area with the sleeping pen inside it. Feed your pup in the pen and have a play with the pup to give the area good associations. Then leave it with a nylon, scented bone to play with. Some people feel that it is cruel to confine a pup in a small area while they are out, but the pup outside, with little to stimulate it, will sleep for a very long time and feels much more secure in a small area. It is certainly preferable to the emotional damage you do by coming home angry.

If you have been careful to develop the right associations with the pen, the pup will not scream when it is put in this area. If, however, you use isolation as a form of punishment, the pup will resent this treatment and soon let you know vocally.

# DISCIPLINE:
# A FEW RULES FOR THE OWNER

Physical punishment is useless in training a dog. The old remedy of the rolled-up newspaper will make the pup cease to trust you and reluctant to come when called. It may even behave aggressively when cornered.

Dogs are creatures of habit, so if you develop good habits from the start, it soon becomes routine for the pup. Adopting a rigid time routine can make a rod for your back however. Dogs may not wear watches but their internal clocks are deadly accurate. If, for example, you develop a habit of taking a dog for a walk at exactly the same time each day, then it will grow up to pester you at that time with tail wags, whines, head-butting and bringing the lead. You will have no peace until you give in and go for a walk.

# PLAYTIME: NOT ALL FUN AND GAMES

Play is for outside, not inside, because pups, like children, get their moments when they want to go mad, which is when accidents happen and something gets broken. Children out of control inside the house always have the same effect, with someone or something getting hurt. Pups need to let off steam as it is all part of their natural development. Call them or carry them outside if they start going mad in the house.

Let the tumbling, rolling and running take its natural course without too much interference as most human intervention results in overstimulation for a dog. If you are instigating the play, let it be in the form of throwing the nylon scented bone. Do not hold the bone in the air to make the pup jump up after it. This is not only bad for the pup's bones, but also teaches it to leap up at moving objects when it is older. These games develop a very strong awareness in a dog of the power of its own mouth, which can too easily turn to biting. Pups do not come with an on–off switch; if rough play is commenced, a pup will become overexcited and hard to control. As the pup grows up it will be able to run rings around you and start uncontrollable rough play whenever it wants. Another way inadvertently to make a pup turn aggressive later in life is to play tug-of-war games, holding-the-muzzle games, or slapping playfully around the mouth, which is courting disaster.

Many owners complain that their pup continually tries to bite their hands without any encouragement from them. Biting your hands is the only way a pup knows to hold your hand. It is a direct attention-getting gesture that must be stopped straight away. The pup should always wear a light collar and, if it goes for your hands, grasp this collar and shake the puppy, saying 'No' several times. Immediately then give a reassuring pat when the shock of what you have done stops the naughty behaviour. In this way you will not cause any bad side effects. The young are always impressionable, so learning through intimidation has become the course in human life, first with parents, then teachers, policemen and bank

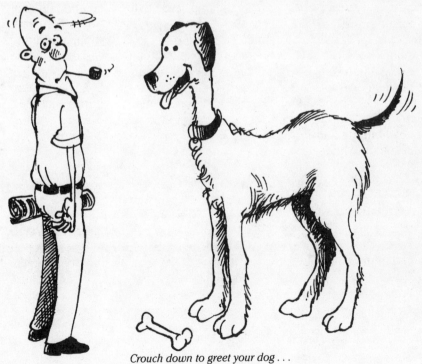

*Crouch down to greet your dog . . .*

managers! The intimidation you use to discipline your pup must be very controlled, however, so that the pup is not permanently suppressed.

Another facet of play to be avoided is encouraging the pup to jump up on you. This may be fine as a greeting when it is young but when it grows to maybe 50 kilograms and you are all dressed up for an evening out, you will not welcome it. So in play greeting, crouch down to the pup's level and fondle it while it is in the sitting position.

You can expect that your dog's character, at the age of 4 months, is well on the way to being shaped if the dog has been exposed to enough experiences. Good habits should have developed with occasional lapses and the dog is ready for formal training.

# 7

# How to Survive Your Pup Aged 4-6 Months

## THE 'TEENAGE' PERIOD

The 4-month-old puppy will be quite receptive to training and yet will not retain everything. Most training classes do not take dogs before age 6 months but some training and control is necessary during this time so that the pup does not become pack-leader of your family. At 4 months, some hormone activity will be taking place, although dogs are not sexually mature until about 10 months or more. This hormone activity can be concurrent with the development of aggression in a dog. For exactly this reason, it is important to let the pup of 4–6 months know who is boss.

Some breeds are wrongly termed 'neurotic' because they indulge in unpredictable behaviour until 2 or even 2½ years old but in fact these are simply late-maturing breeds such as Labradors, Afghan hounds and Old English sheepdogs, to mention only a few. One can liken these dogs to a teenage girl who will display all the wiles of womanhood and a maturity beyond her years, only suddenly to transform into a little girl having a terrible temper tantrum, which can leave some parents feeling mentally battered and bewildered. Something of the same parental authority, tempered with love and understanding, is needed to control your dog at this tender age.

# 'DON'T INVADE MY SPACE': CRITICAL DISTANCE

In your dealings with your pup at this age you will become very aware of the *critical distance*. I get a lot of fun watching people in the park with their dogs, especially when they don't have a clue what they are dealing with. The scenario usually goes something like this: the pup is bounding around enjoying itself in close proximity to the owner when, as it moves a little further away, the owner calls it. The pup almost imperceptibly creeps off a bit further before making a wild dash. The owner rushes after it yelling for it to come back, but the pup is now in full flight! This is where teaching to recall on a long leash increases the critical distance between dog and owner and allows you to get the dog to come when called.

We all have an area of personal territory around us that we do not like to be invaded by strangers and if, at a party for example, someone comes up too close whom we do not like, then we back away. The area of personal territory around a dog is usually about 1½ metres. A scared dog, whom you are trying to coax to come to you, stays outside this radius. Your own pup will also run rings around you staying just outside the 1½-metre limit. It will tease you mercilessly, bounding around playfully just out of reach so you cannot catch it. You feel silly, you look sillier and this can provoke anger and yelling. But then, no dog in its right mind is going to come back to a yelling owner!

I once saw a Maltese dart quick as a flash out of a Mercedes Benz without its owner noticing its escape. A weighty lady, balancing precariously on stiletto heels, got out of the car and saw the Maltese making off. She tottered off in pursuit with her voice gradually reaching a shrieking pitch. Back went the pup's ears, down went its head and off it shot faster than ever, this time in fear-inspired flight. I never did catch up with the end of that episode; for all I know, they may still be running!

To avoid this situation, get that early recall training really consolidated and if the teenage pup is showing reluctance to come, then train it on a long leash. This needs to be about 10 metres in length, or you can buy a retractable lead that gets less tangled up. Coax the pup to you from a short distance at first, then gradually increase the distance until eventually you can achieve the same success off the leash. Reward or praise the pup when it comes to you but *never* yell at it to come or hit your dog once you have caught it, as this is the most efficient way to teach a dog to never come when it is called.

# EARLY TRAINING: 'DO-IT-YOURSELF'

At age 4–6 months it is time to have a crack at training the pup yourself, as most formal classes do not take pups until they are 6 months old. Now is the time to buy a choke-chain. Slip the chain through one of the bigger rings, which are at each end, to form a collar. Put it over the pup's head so that when the pup is on leash beside you, on your left side, the ring to which it is attached slides along the chain freely. If you have it on upside down, the chain locks when you pull it so that, even when the pressure is taken off, the chain does not release. It is very easy to check that you have the choke-chain on correctly, simply by trial and error.

With the pup on your left side, walk forward with the leash held in the left hand, fairly near to the pup, and the end of the leash in the right hand. If the pup pulls ahead, a short jerk on the leash, across your body, accompanied by the word 'heel' should pull the pup back into line. Do not maintain pressure on the chain but release it immediately. If the choke-chain is used harshly, the pup will become stressed.

For bumptious characters who forge ahead, pulling hard on the chain and determined to fight it, do lots of left- and right-hand turns. Turn left by pulling back on the lead to bring the pup back into line and turn right by turning with a slack lead. The pup then learns that the

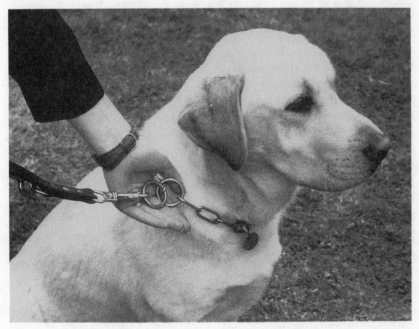

*Make sure you put the choke-chain on the right way up.*

most comfortable place for it to be is just behind you on your left side. For some dogs that are too boisterous, or that make your arms nearly pop out of their sockets, get one of Dr Roger Mugford's halters. Dr Mugford, a well-known animal behaviourist from the United Kingdom, has transferred the simple principle of guiding from the head, used in the world of horses, to the training of dogs. After all, who ever heard of a horse wearing a choke-chain? They come in sizes from 0 to 5 with different widths. I once saw a flighty Great Dane being led successfully on one of these halters by a child and this same dog had given his owners hell on a choke-chain.

After mastering the walking at heel, you can progress to 'sit'. Pull the lead up and back and, with your other hand on the dog's rump, push the dog down to the sitting position, accompanied by the word 'sit'. Dogs and owners proudly show off this stunt but it is amusing to see most dogs, after 'obediently' sitting, immediately popping straight back up again! To get them used to sitting without getting up straight away, circle them from right to left and vice versa with the lead above their head. They are so busy watching you that they forget to stand up. If dogs are to be shown in the ring, then you are not supposed to train them to 'sit' by a push down on the rump because when the judge handles them by running a hand down their back they will automatically go to the 'sit' position instead of standing at attention.

Getting a dog to go down in the lying position is hard, because it means you are being strongly dominant. It is usually achieved from the 'sit' position by placing the dog down by the front legs. None of this training is as easy as it seems, which is why it is best to get professional help. You will read more about that in Chapter 15 (page 172), which describes types of training. Some people, however, cannot get professional lessons or simply don't want to. To successfully train a dog by yourself, you have to be calm, confident, assertive but not bullying and have limitless patience. I am a hopeless trainer myself and leave it to Jim's expertise. If you're lucky, of course, you might have a dog that is what we call a 'natural'; it seems to sense what you want and just does it. If so, you will be the envy of all dog owners!

PART III

# Health Care

# 8

# First Visit to the Vet

Your first trip to the vet with your pup will probably be for its vaccination shots a few days after it has settled in with you. This is usually at about 6 weeks of age, if the breeder has not already arranged to have the pup given the first set of shots. A little commonsense and sensitivity on your part can avoid turning this initial encounter with the vet into a traumatic experience for both you and your dog.

Before you leave home for the vet's, make your pup go to the toilet in the garden. Once you are in the vet's waiting room keep your pup in your arms because, although the surgery floor has probably had a disinfectant wash that morning, you never know what animal patients may come in carrying something infectious.

So far, so good. When it is your turn, you go into the surgery and put your pup on the table. Now is the moment of truth and this is what usually happens. If it has been properly socialised, the pup will be playing happily on the surgery table. I make a habit of loading the syringe with my back to the pup so it can't see it. Dogs have excellent memories and they never forget the sight of a syringe. Unfortunately, however, the owner has usually seen the syringe. Our perfectly contented puppy suddenly changes into a shaking, wrinkle-browed, pathetic little heap. Why this dramatic change of mood?

The owner, who is scared stiff of needles, has immediately conveyed his own fear to the pup through his anxious tone of voice and body language. He immediately snuggles the puppy up close and cossets and soothes it with a sympathetic, crooning voice so that the

111

pup instantly suspects something terrible is about to happen to it.

Mothers inadvertently do the same thing with their children. A mother will rush over to her toddler who has taken a tumble on the grass and the child, although quite unhurt, will react to its mother's face, contorted with panic and concern, by bursting into tears. Another mum in the same circumstances will laugh and say jokingly 'My! You made a big dent in the ground and woke up a gnome having a snooze!' The child will continue playing happily, unconcerned about the fall or the rudely awakened gnome.

So act cheerfully with your pup and the needle will be over before you know it while you and the vet are carrying on a normal conversation. Most vets pop the shots under the skin in the neck region; this is called a subcutaneous injection.

If the pup is large and boisterous and needs restraint, do not grab hold of it tightly because most pups will immediately panic and fight your grip. Hold it close to your body with one arm around its neck so it cannot see the syringe and the other arm cuddled over its back. By holding an animal in a natural position like this you do not upset it and the needle is easier to insert when there is no struggle or resistance.

My advice to owners to stay light and cheerful while we are giving their dog an injection generally works very well although some owners have been known to start cooing maternally in the middle of the operation and ruin the whole thing. There was one memorable lady, however, who did not quite understand what I intended or, if she did, her approach went terribly wrong.

This particular client swept into the surgery one day with a diminutive but overindulged silkie that bit whenever and whatever it wanted, worse than any other dog I had met.

'There, there, my poor little darling,' the woman shrieked in a voice of doom as if the bomb was about to drop, 'of course you are very frightened.'

'Perhaps you could be a little quieter,' I suggested tactfully. 'He is only getting scared because of the frightened tone of your own voice. Just laugh, chat, sing if you like, to reassure him that everything is all right.'

She did. I did not anticipate her full-blast rendition of a Wagnerian operatic aria. Nor did the dog! It promptly went berserk and as the aria reached its ear-splitting tragic climax, she jigged the poor animal up and down to 'calm' him. 'Goodness,' I thought as I tried to soothe the savage beast, 'I hope she never has any grandchildren!'

The right approach for the first time at the vet will save endless trouble when you next visit. I have well-adjusted patients who run into the surgery and jump up on the table all by themselves, depositing a big, wet 'kiss' on my face. There are others, however, who, even when just out for a walk near my surgery, will madly drag their owners to the opposite side of the road risking death under the wheels of a lorry to escape! Happily, these dogs are the exceptions.

## BRIBERY AND BLACKMAIL: A TWO-WAY GAME

Bribery may be a bad general principle for raising dogs (and children) but the odd doggy chocolate, proffered to a patient who is not off its food, works wonders. As a rule, owners should not encourage dogs to accept food from strangers so I use this method with discretion – and the owner's permission of course! As a vet, I think 'baby talk' is permissable too as a way of reassuring an animal because I know for a fact that most owners do exactly the same thing when they think nobody is listening.

Use 'baby talk' with caution however. For example, using an over-sympathetic voice with a dog who has suffered a minor injury that leaves him with a temporary limp can often produce so-called 'sympathy lameness'. As a result, a perfectly healthy dog will learn to affect a limp to get your undivided attention. Similarly, a dog who has been over-protected during its first thunderstorm will freak out at every thunderstorm for the rest of its life.

My experience of dog owners 'mothering' their animals makes me wonder who ever accused men of not being nurturing creatures? Men are big sooks when it comes to dogs and they cluck and coo as much as any woman who is supposedly sublimating her maternal instincts by 'babying' a pup.

Be warned: dogs are masterful in gaining sympathy and attention. Even as I write this sentence, my dog is busily chewing off the bottom of his pad while eyeing me closely to make sure I have noticed. I know there is absolutely nothing wrong with his foot but that if he goes on chewing it there soon will be. Obviously he is bored and thinks he is overdue for a walk. This time he's got the better of me. Even we vets are not impervious to those sooky feelings that dogs are so clever at arousing in their owners.

# 9

# Vaccinations

John Mainwaring fixed me with a glinting look. 'I sometimes wonder if you vets are taking us for a ride. I've never heard of distemper these days, so I quite frankly question if all these vaccinations are necessary?' he said accusingly. His 3-month-old bull terrier looked up at him with its humorous piggy little eyes as if in thorough agreement.

'Only the other day,' I began to explain, 'a young man with an art gallery brought in his 13-year-old dog, who was in splendid bodily condition and had a potential longevity of at least 18 years I'd say, and looked no more than about 8 years old. The only problem was that he was showing abnormal neurological symptoms, standing in corners, falling over and not recognising his owner. On investigation, this behaviour turned out to be caused by post-distemper encephalitis. The owner was heartbroken. He had not realised that regular vaccinations were necessary, and somehow never got beyond believing the "one needle for life was enough".'

'Well it *was* the case when I was a boy,' replied John, stroking his beard thoughtfully. 'The problem is that now there is more public awareness,' I continued, 'so more dogs are vaccinated and as a result there is less "street" virus around to boost their immunity naturally while they are still protected by their first needles. This is the reason why annual vaccinations have become necessary. To stop regularly vaccinating dogs would be akin to what might happen if we stopped vaccinating our children against polio.'

'OK you win!' he said. Bongo, his ally, just stood there stoically like a typical bull terrier and didn't even realise he'd already had his vaccination shot while we talked!

# DISEASES FOR WHICH THERE ARE VACCINATIONS

## Distemper

The start of distemper in a dog is insidious, with no more to show than a fever for a few days. The non-observant owner may easily miss that their dog is sick. The dog may even appear to have fully recovered from the sickness but in a few days the eyes and nose will begin to discharge and this later turns to heavy yellow pus. Then the dog won't eat and often develops pneumonia. Much of the infection by this time is secondary bacterial, where non-viral germs have leapt into the dog's system due to the dog's lowered resistance. Antibiotics can therefore be of some benefit, as can vitamins, especially the B group, although the viral part of the disease will have to run its course.

Even after apparent recovery, the owner will suffer cliff-hanging suspense for weeks, waiting to see if the dog develops post-distemper

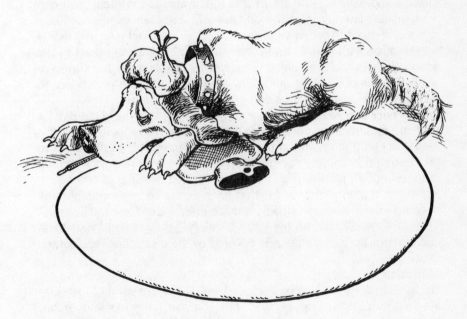

*'Sick as a dog' can be very real.*

encephalitis. This condition can be in the form of chorea, where groups of muscles twitch with relentless spasms even when the dog is asleep. There may develop a drunken stagger in the back legs, fits or even a total change of personality where the dog you once knew and trusted will be in a highly nervous state and will bite you and not recognise who you are. Distemper, once diagnosed, need not be a death sentence but when the nervous symptoms have developed, the chances of recovery are narrowed down to almost nil. Sometimes the odd case where fits have occurred or some cases of chorea will recover or be left with just a weakness.

### Vaccinations

Many people query why they have to go to the vet for distemper, hepatitis and parvovirus vaccinations at age about 6–8 weeks and at 12–14 weeks. The reason is because there is no cheap and easy way to measure just how much immunity, in the form of antibodies, the mother dog bestowed upon her puppies in the first milk, or colostrum, to use the correct term. These antibodies block the vaccine from taking. By age 3 months, however, they are all eliminated from the pup's system. If the mother's immunity was not strong and the antibodies are rapidly eliminated from the pup's system, you may well end up with a pup who is walking about totally unprotected.

Then why can't you keep the pup isolated, or 'quarantined', until 3 months and save on one set of shots? The risk is too great. You can walk inside, carrying infection on your feet. Your fences are not likely to be 'sniff-proof'. Another vital factor to consider is that your pup needs socialisation with people and other dogs, and it must get used to the scary things in the everyday environment, such as a car backfiring or a neighbour's dog acting out a territorial fence-ritual of pretending to be very fierce. You can't lock up your pup for 3 months.

Even with vaccine protection, your pup will be at some slight risk for the first 3 months so do not let it mix with any dogs who appear unhealthy. Also don't let it sniff around lamp-posts and trees. It is fun for dogs to go through this sniffing routine in order to see who was there before them as a dog's nose acts as its telly, radio and newspaper combined, but there is plenty of time for that later. Some people actually think having a dog on a lead is a magic 'germ barrier' – don't fall into this trap!

In the United Kingdom the virus 'hard pad', not present in Australia and first cousin to distemper, is covered by the distemper vaccination.

### Hepatitis

Hepatitis in dogs is not to be confused with human hepatitis. Most dogs are immune after the first year of life but if they are going to shows or they belong to breeders or are being boarded they should be regularly vaccinated because of their exposure to so many dogs. Hepatitis is a virus that hits the liver. Death can be sudden and symptomless or there may be warning signs of nausea, vomiting and depression. Never attempt a home diagnosis but see your vet at the slightest sign of any sickness.

## Parvovirus

This disease struck worldwide in 1978 and the death toll was enormous, with no respect for strength, sex or age. The symptoms are vomiting, acute depression, and passing of foul-smelling diarrhoea that looks like port wine. Death can be rapid. These cases need emergency treatment and hospitalisation with the dog put on an intravenous drip of life-supporting fluids and treated with other therapy while the virus takes its course. The virus can affect the heart muscle in pups, which causes a sudden, rapid and very distressing death but no other symptoms.

### Vaccinations

To prevent parvovirus two initial vaccinations are necessary at 6–8 weeks and 12–14 weeks and sometimes at 6 months. The length of time between boosters, that is to say, repeat vaccinations, varies according to the particular country and circumstances, so be guided by your vet, although annual vaccinations are usual in Australia.

## Leptospirosis

Leptospirosis is a bacterial infection that can be transmitted to humans. It is nearly always caught where there are rats, although other animals can act as carriers. The main source of infection is water infected with animal urine. The disease can affect the liver and kidneys; fever, vomiting and jaundice are the main symptoms. Pets in Australia are not usually vaccinated against this disease.

## Kennel cough

This cough is a real 'graveyard cough', hacking and deep-seated. It is not a wet, soft kind of cough but one that shakes the very guts. A coughing bout is often followed by gagging and bringing up mucus. As the name suggests, the condition can be a big problem in boarding kennels and veterinary hospitals due to the very infectious nature of the virus; it has no connection with the cleanliness of the kennels. It was affectionately known in London many years ago as 'Battersea Dogs' Home cough'. You can, however, get outbreaks among the general dog population and, although it can occur at any age, it usually affects only young dogs. Kennel cough is not a killer disease and there is rarely fever. The cause is viral and the disease can be complicated by secondary bacterial infection, although a bacterium, *Bordetella bronchiseptica*, may be the only cause in some cases.

When Mrs Stokes's pup had kennel cough, she said to me, 'You know, that cough sounds terrifying to me. Why, if my husband had it he would think he was dying yet Tara couldn't care less. She is tearing around the garden as if there was nothing wrong with her!' Kennel cough can last up to about six weeks and just has to take its course. The dog should remain fairly quiet and the temperature of its environment should be kept as even as possible. Antibiotics can be of some use against the bacterial side of the infection.

Owners are very tempted to use human cough suppressants for dogs with this condition but a cough has a purpose, which is to get up mucus and inflammatory products clogging the respiratory tract. Dosing a dog with cough medicine will only make this mucus stay put and this makes matters much worse. Of course there are some coughs that have become so tickly that a little cough sedation may be helpful, but only administer after veterinary advice.

*Vaccinations*
There is a vaccine available against the virus. Two doses four weeks apart should protect young pups for a year but, as it is not a killer virus, vaccinations are not strictly necessary. To protect your adult dog in boarding kennels, one dose of vaccine ten days beforehand will protect it.

**Rabies**
'Mad dogs and Englishmen go out in the midday sun,' goes the refrain of Noel Coward's famous song, reminiscent of all those old raj stories along the theme, 'Poor chap he was bitten by a mad dog in India, you know!' Rabies is the most 'celebrated' of the animal diseases and the dreaded rabies virus is deservedly so. It attacks the nervous system, taking up to one year to incubate, and recovery is almost nil.

Although the virus is worldwide, Australia and the United Kingdom have kept rabies at bay so far because of their strict quarantine policies and the fact that they are islands. Countries with no sea 'barriers' are at great risk as animals can easily slip across borders, as in the case of a cat from India who arrived at quarantine in Holland. Not only was the poor creature rabid but its cage had a false bottom in which was concealed hashish. The cat had been set up as a drug smuggler but no one had bothered to check its health! Wildlife acts as a reservoir for the virus and the particular carrier may display no symptoms. In the United States, for example, foxes, bats, skunks and raccoons are common carriers.

In the 'furious' type of rabies, a dog may show a change of temperament and go 'sooky' or 'mad'; it may wander and bite at moving objects and may appear to feel no pain. In the other form, 'dumb' rabies, the dog may become paralysed and dribble saliva; this latter form can occur alone or as a sequel to furious rabies.

## Vaccinations

Rabies shots are compulsory in the United States and all vaccinated dogs must wear tags to prove they are protected. They are first vaccinated at age 3–4 months and then at about a year, with boosters every few years, although this varies in some states. No vaccinations are required in Australia, New Zealand or the United Kingdom because of their tight quarantine rules that have, to date, kept the disease from their shores.

## Essential vaccinations

These are distemper, hepatitis and parvovirus shots at age 6–8 weeks and 12–14 weeks, and sometimes a further parvovirus at age 6 months. From then on annual vaccinations are necessary.

Always check with your vet about the latest vaccine programme as research is being carried out all the time.

# 10

# Puppy Care

Mrs Fitzsimmons's toy poodle only half-viewed the world through a cascading top-knot of hair. For the same reason, Mrs Fitzsimmons had only a half-view of her dog's eyes so that when he got a bad case of conjunctivitis, she had not noticed the condition until the damage had got to the deeper layers of the corneas and the dog's vision was permanently impaired. This sad result could have been prevented if Mrs Fitzsimmons had checked her dog's eyes regularly. Just like the regular oil and grease change in a car, routine maintenance prevents a lot of other things going wrong.

Learning to cast your eye expertly over your pup on a regular basis can save the animal a lot of unnecessary suffering and stop any damage to your pocket-nerve also. Instead of a dictionary of hundreds of ailments, this section will serve as an easy-to-read puppy maintenance guide that should prevent any of the really big nasties occurring.

## BRUSHING AND BATHING

Brushing does wonders. It stimulates the dog's skin circulation to promote a shiny coat and the loose hair and dust that comes out in a good brushing won't be dropped all over your house. Brushing short-coated dogs is fine with a soft bristle brush but longer coats may need special grooming tools such as wire brushes. Plenty of brushing means that you can cut down on bathing your dog. This is desirable because bathing, if overdone, can wash all the natural oil out of a dog's coat and cause dryness and itching. The natural oil in the coat already has some cleansing qualities and the more you bath a dog the more frequently you end up having to do it.

If fleas are around, it's best to only use a shampoo with pyrethrum, which discourages fleas but is safe for the pup. If the pup has no fleas, a mild shampoo will do but use a doggy formula shampoo as it has the correct pH balance so that the pup's skin does not become irritated. Human shampoos often have perfume, which can cause the dog's skin to tickle. There are also doggy hair-conditioners for long, tangled coats.

Get a pup used to being bathed while it is still young or later on it will act as if it is a prisoner on the run, discreetly disappearing whenever it sees dog-bath preparations in motion. Some dogs just hate being bathed. They become shaking, nervous wrecks before their bath and then cavort like pups afterwards with the relief of it all being over. A favourite doggy trick is to immediately go and roll in the manure on the rose bed so you end up right back at square one.

Some of the things that promote fear of bath-time are water that is too hot or too cold, hoses that hit them full blast, and the scary noise of taps running while they are in the tub. With small pups, prepare the tub before putting them in and take them out again when you want to replace the water for rinsing.

Large pups and big dogs often have to be bathed tied up on the ground, using a bucket of warm water and a hosing off to finish. This means picking a day when a cold wind is not blowing. Always make sure to rinse very thoroughly otherwise many dogs go into a severe scratching session afterwards. Take care also to wipe the dog's face with a flannel instead of showering it with water, which dogs hate. Do not let water get in the ears or soap get in the eyes.

After the bath, put the dog in a warm, draught-free place to dry. Do not bath a pup if it has just had its vaccinations. On the other hand, a bath the day before desexing will be greatly appreciated by the vet, whose assistant has to prepare the operation site so that it is germ-free.

The general rule is only bath your dog when it is dirty and not as a routine. There are some dogs who just love to roll in faeces and dead wildlife. The reason is not totally clear but it seems it's their way of gaining allure, the equivalent if you like of wearing Chanel No. 5 and maybe associated in some obscure way with instincts to disguise their own scent from an enemy. Try to find the offending dead smelly creature and then dispose of it as the first thing that your dog will want to do after its bath is go straight back and with fanatic compulsion roll in the carcass all over again! Rolling in rottenness seems to promote confidence; dogs always look very pleased with themselves afterwards.

On one occasion my Weimaraner looked incredibly smug after he had rolled in human excreta. His joy somewhat abated when we had to tie him in the back of our stationwagon in such a way that he could not move or lie down. He was also wrapped in an old rug that never saw the light of day again. After being blasted at long distance on the pavement with the hose on full, he and I did not speak for days!

# PEDICURE

Many pups have dew claws, which are a dog's equivalent to thumbs, situated on the inside of the leg just above the foot, and may or may not have a pad. These claws can be on the back or front legs and sometimes the claw is placed in such a way that it will grow, curling around and wending its way right into the pad, causing a nasty infected sore. This can easily be missed in long-haired dogs.

The dew claws should be kept trimmed at all times. They are often surgically removed in pups a few days old or in older dogs when they are undergoing surgery for something else such as desexing. I see no point in removing these claws if they are causing no trouble. Some stick out more than others, however, and, often in the case of working dogs, they will catch and tear. Should that happen, they should of course be removed (see page 132). Dogs who take some of their exercise on roads

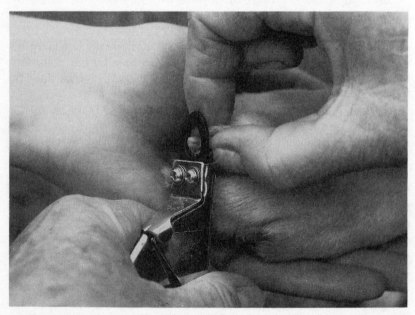

*Hold the nail between your fingers and avoid the pink blood vessel at the nail when cutting.*

or have a concrete area in their yard will usually wear their nails down but those dogs who run only on soft ground often get long nails that need clipping. Nails can also grow too long in dogs that have flat feet, as the nail is not contacting the ground and being thus worn down.

To keep your dog's nails trimmed, invest in a good-quality pair of guillotine clippers. Unlike the name suggests, you can do a painless nail cut with these as they do not transfer pressure up the nail to sensitive nerves as do ordinary nail clippers. If the pup has white nails it is easy to see the pink blood vessel through the nail. Avoid cutting this as the resulting trauma will produce a dog that freaks out every time it has its nails cut. Some dogs snatch their foot away when you are trying to cut their nails. Get someone to hold the dog for you, cuddling it up against them with one arm around the neck, so the dog cannot see what you are doing, and the other hand behind the elbow so that the leg is in a lock. Then you can hold the nail between thumb and first finger, which seems to stop pain transferring up the nail. Usually it is easier to cut a dog's back nails as it cannot see what is going on! Some dogs who fight as if for their very life will stand quite quietly if you cut the nails with the foot on the ground in the natural standing position.

# EAR CARE

## Wax
The expression 'If it ain't broke, don't fix it' applies very well to the care of a dog's ears. Look inside regularly to see if there is any wax, which in dogs is dark brown. Long-eared breeds such as bassets are particularly prone to excess wax, which can cause irritation, scratching and secondary infection. The wax can also block the ear and cause partial deafness. See your vet if the pup has wax. Many owners cause damage to their dog's ears by cleaning them out with orange sticks, rubbing the delicate lining and maybe going too deep near the eardrum.

## Drops
Gone are the days of a 'cure-all' medication for ears where every bottle of drops contained drugs for bacteria, fungi, yeasts, as well as wax removers, local anaesthetics and cortisone as an anti-inflammatory ingredient. Using these drops, a 'miraculous' cure followed after a couple of days – the result was a happy owner and a happy vet! Then the whole trouble recurred a month or so later until the treatment finally ceased to work. Why? Because drug-resistant strains of infection have set up in the ear and then you are really in trouble. Swelling causes the opposite sides of the ear canal to rub together, resulting in ulcers that are excruciatingly painful for the dog. Then an operation is necessary to open

up the canal so that the sides do not rub and air can circulate, but even this does not always totally solve the problem.

If an owner regularly checks a dog's ears, such a situation need never arise. Nowadays your vet will give you eardrops that do not sting and that will work the wax up by itself, so all you have to do is wipe it away with a piece of water-dampened, squeezed-out cotton wool on your finger – not on the end of a stick.

### Seeds

Country dogs often get grass seeds down their ears, causing a head-standing, mind-bursting tickle. The onset is sudden and the vet should be seen as soon as possible; grass seeds left down the ear can cause long-term chronic ear problems.

### Mites

Especially with dogs who sleep in close proximity to cats, ear mites can be a problem. Invisible to the naked eye, these creepy-crawlies, often buried in wax, cause a tickle by doing a dance down the ear canal. This condition can be diagnosed with the microscope and the vet will prescribe suitable drops.

### Haemorrhage in the earflap

This causes it to swell up like a balloon, and usually only occurs in older dogs who have some chronic ear trouble. Plagued by a bad ear, they shake their heads a lot, rupturing one of the ear's tiny blood vessels. Surgery is usually needed in such a case, but often hirudoid ointment, a favourite for bruised footballers, will clear the blood clot.

### Local allergic reaction

Sometimes the bare underside of the earflap becomes irritated by something in the environment such as grasses and goes red and hot. The dog shakes its head because of the irritation and may start trouble further down the ear. Wash the flaps, without getting water down the ear, just to remove the irritation and cover the affected area with pawpaw ointment or vaseline to act as a physical barrier to the irritant. This treatment is often enough to arrest the condition. Some irritations of the earflap are caused by food allergy or fatty acid deficiency.

### Signs of ear problems

Head-shaking, rubbing the ear along the ground or scratching it are usually the first signs of ear problems in a dog. The more chronic case will hold its head to one side or hold the ear flattened against the head. Any bad smell coming from the ear spells trouble. Also, any yellow discharge should be regarded very seriously and requires an immediate

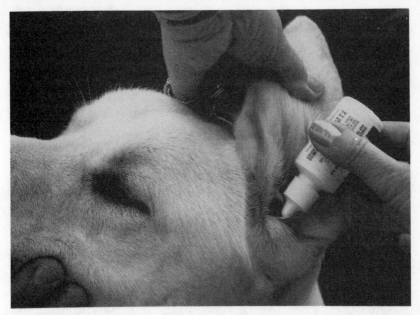

*Hold the ear vertically so the eardrops reach the bottom of the ear canal.*

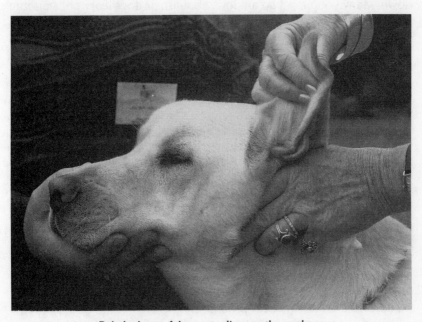

*Rub the base of the ear to disperse the eardrops.*

visit to the vet. Remember though that in some bad ear cases there are no early signs so you must always do a regular check.

### Putting in eardrops

Sometimes ears do not get better under treatment because owners do not put the drops or ointment in correctly. They often flatten the ear across the top of the head so the ear canal closes and the drops do not go to the bottom where they are needed. If you hold the ear up vertically by the tip, this opens up the canal so the drops hit the spot. Then you should massage the base of the ear where you will hear a squelching sound, indicating the drops have collected in the right place. Of course, some dog's ears feel 'squelchy' anyway. This is a sure sign that there is discharge in the ear due to excess wax or infection. Take appropriate action.

### One up, one down

Owners of some pedigree dogs, whose ears are supposed to be erect, go through weeks of anxiety when instead their dogs' ears just flop. This condition is often due to teething as it seems the local pain in the mouth causes the muscles that make the ears stand up to not function properly. Some pups' ears can end up in a bizarre position where they are so erect that they cross over while others end up with one ear up and one down. Many people get so anxious about their dogs' ears not standing up, they even try fastening them in place with tape. This is totally ineffective. If the ears are not going to become normal again, you might as well forget about it. Of course if those ears do not end up in the right place, it may spoil you pup's chances for the show ring, but it does not detract from the health of the pup, which is really all that matters.

# TOOTH CARE

### Mouth-shy

Sleepless nights spent with a teething baby is par for the course for parents of a human infant so count yourself lucky you are spared the same problem with pups. Pups do go through a stage of teething problems, which is when they will become particularly mouthy and chew anything and everything. Pups may also become fractious when you handle their mouths, and accidently touch their gums, for example, in the process of worming. Great care should be taken to be gentle during this time, otherwise they could become 'mouth-shy' and dosing by mouth will then always be a problem.

Pups grow one set of baby teeth, which they then shed until they have a completely new set by the age of about 8 months. Quite often a pup will be left with a double set of canines, or 'fang' teeth, which are the ones used for grabbing and tearing, unlike the big back molars used for grinding food. The front incisors are never very developed as they are not important teeth in carnivores: they do not need them for chomping grass as do sheep and cattle. Double canines are uncomfortable and come about because the second set of teeth did not push the first baby teeth out as they erupted. Look out for this in your pup at about age 5–6 months. Sometimes a coin rocked between the two new teeth will loosen the old one but do not attempt this if it upsets the pup. Leave the problem to the vet.

### A dog's toothbrush?

Although it is highly unlikely that your pup will gather tartar on the teeth until it is much older, it makes good sense to get it used to having its teeth cleaned once it has completed teething and its sore gums have settled down at about 9 or 10 months. Penny, a 10-year-old toy poodle, quite happily accepts her owner cleaning her teeth weekly with her own electric toothbrush and powdered toothpaste.

This teeth-cleaning habit prevents the build-up of tartar into hard hunks that the vet has to then clean off, giving the dog an anaesthetic. If you are not into gadgets, then an ordinary soft toothbrush and a paste

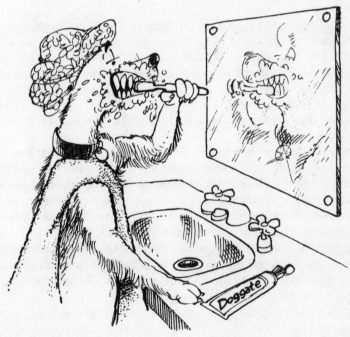

*Specially angulated toothbrushes and non-foaming toothpastes are available.*

of bicarbonate of soda will do; some dogs hate toothpaste so bicarbonate of soda does the trick and, if swallowed, produces nothing more than a burp.

People often laugh at the thought of cleaning dogs' teeth, probably because most people don't kiss dogs on the mouth. Nevertheless, 85 per cent of dogs over the age of 3 years have problems with teeth and gums, and this can easily be prevented. North American veterinary surgeons pioneered preventative dental treatment for dogs and as a result toothbrushes with suitable angulation can now be obtained as well as a non-foaming toothpaste that contains an enzyme system designed to kill the bacteria that cause plaque. For dogs who will not accept brushing there is a bone-shaped, grooved, rubber toy that massages the gums. By smoothing paste onto the toy, the paste works it way into tooth crevices and cleans the dog's teeth with no need for brushing. There are gauze pads with a similar action for the reluctant patient.

Not only does tooth care help your pet's health; it makes life much pleasanter for the dog owner by eliminating the need for nicknames such as 'death-breath', as one of my patients is not so affectionately called!

# EYE CARE

**Problem eyes**
Even if you purchased a clear, bright-eyed pup with no weeping or apparent irritation, it is just possible that inherited defects will not make themselves known until well after you have made your selection or purchase. Eyelids may roll in, causing irritation. This is most common in the Great Dane, golden retriever, Irish setter, chow chow, St Bernard, bulldog and Chesapeake Bay retriever. It can be corrected surgically by taking a small crescent-shaped fold out of the lid, which pulls it away from the eye.

In other breeds the lids may roll out to give a somewhat drunken, red-eyed appearance. St Bernards and some of the hounds are most affected by this condition. Extra eyelashes or short, stubby ones that point the wrong way may occur and cause rubbing on the eyes. Any breed can be affected by this but it is most common in poodles, spaniels and Pekingese. These conditions can be fixed by surgery.

Deep skin folds on the faces of breeds such as bulldogs and Pekingese encourage bacterial infection in the folds. This can lead in turn to eye infections that cause conjunctivitis and even deeper infections in the cornea, the thick outside layer of the eyeball.

Beagles, bulldogs, Boston terriers and some other breeds sometimes have a small gland under the third eyelid which is not properly attached and it can pop out from under the lid and cause irritation. (The third eyelid, which plays an important part in cleaning the surface of the eye, comes from the corner of the eye and goes under the two other lids. In most breeds it can only just be seen in the corner of the eye near the nose.) Often this gland becomes enlarged and needs surgical removal. Discharging eyes can be symptomatic of a disease and if you suspect this is so, see the vet immediately. It may be a simple allergy from dust or sprays, but don't take any risks.

### Damage to the eye

Coming out second best in confrontation with a moggy can often result in a damaged eye, especially if your dog doesn't duck a swipe from the cat's claw. Sometimes the wound even penetrates the cornea, which can lead to serious complications, so a vet should be seen straight away. Walking into thorns or protruding wire can result in similar damage. It is, not surprisingly, pop-eyed pups like Pekingese who are most prone to cornea damage of this kind.

If your pup suddenly has eye irritation and one or both of its eyes start to water, or it begins rubbing its eye along the ground or pawing at it, you must treat this as a serious sign and see the vet immediately. Eyes are too precious for you to mess around with home treatments. Although it may well turn out to be only a simple skin irritation or allergy around the eye, never, but never, take the risk of diagnosing eye problems yourself.

## DOSING YOUR DOG

Many owners cannot dose their dogs; some dogs bite, some – like pekes – go purple with fury, others have neck muscles like an ox and jerk their head around. Tablets you thought were down the hatch end up in your eyes or are stealthily disgorged in a corner of the room some time later. Disguising tablets in food with a sniffer such as your dog's won't fool it.

### Giving tablets

Put the dog on a table; this way it has no advantage. Get someone to hold it in the sitting position from behind. Face it and put your left thumb in its mouth behind the fang tooth and tickle the roof; the dog will open its mouth. Then push the tablet down to the back of the throat with the index finger of the other hand. Rub its throat gently. (See page 130.)

### Giving liquid medicine

Pull the pouch out at the corner of the dog's mouth and pour the liquid in slowly with a spoon or it will be blown all over you. Rub the dog's throat gently. Never dose it with its mouth wide open – it's a good way for your dog to drown. (See page 131.)

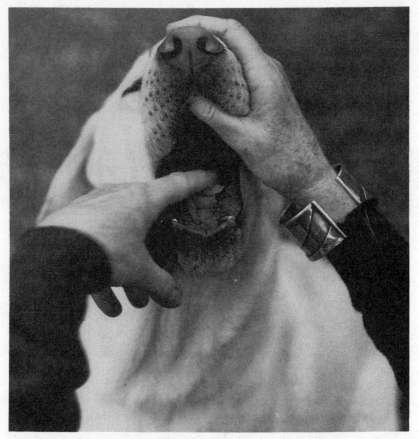

*To give a pill tickle the roof of the mouth with your thumb and push the pill
down with the first finger of the other hand.*

# COSMETIC SURGERY

### Tail docking

If the veterinary profession got its own way there wouldn't be a single
little boy left – well, that's if you believe that little boys are made from
'slugs and snails and puppy dogs' tails'! Because generally speaking
the profession is against tail docking.

A dog was born with a tail for a good reason. It has many different
functions. A tail acts as a rudder in the water. In its native snow country,
a dog like a Siberian Samoyed would sleep at night with its bushy tail
curled over its body and nose to distribute the warm, exhaled air from
its nostrils all over its body to keep it warm. A tail also helps balance
at the run, although some racing greyhounds who for some reason such

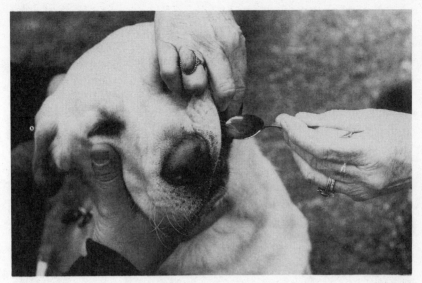

*Give liquid medicine by pulling the pouch out at the corner of the mouth and slowly pouring in the liquid.*

as injury have had their tails docked have still won their races, so speed is not affected. And a tail can tell you much about a dog's mood such as wagging for pleasure.

Tradition dictates that docking is smart and fashionable, and it is the die-hard breeders who are the hardest to convince about the evils of tail docking. They claim that it is not painful; pups cry just as much if their mother steps on them, they say. Of course, they well might – it hurts! Breeders say that pups go straight to their mother to feed off her after docking but this is in fact well-documented displacement behaviour, which indicates pain! So much for the breeders' claims. It is legal, nonetheless, for breeders to dock tails themselves. But the act of tail docking for cosmetic purposes by an unqualified person will be prohibited from 1 July 1993 in the United Kingdom, and as the profession is against docking this means it will be phased out. Tail docking is not without some fatalities. Vets at least usually use a local anaesthetic when they dock and stitch pups' tails at 4 days old.

The shorter the tail is docked, the worse the consequences. The anal sphincter muscles and some small muscles around the anal area are responsible for the anus compressing and shortening during defecation in order to facilitate the process. These muscles have complex attachments down the tail which, if cut, cause less rectal muscle tone and lead to a build-up of faeces in the colon. This fact accounts for the high incidence of hernias lateral to the tail, that is, perineal hernia in dogs with docked tails. Also dogs like corgis, traditionally docked very close to the body, are incredibly 'tail conscious', often biting at the rear end as if experiencing nerve pain. The European convention for the protection of pet animals, under article 10, calls for the procedure to be banned. The Australian Veterinary Association is also against docking. Once dogs start winning in the show ring with undocked tails, the tide of prejudice will turn. In my practice, two pedigree breeders have ceased docking and there are some happy long-tailed cocker spaniels and schnauzers as a result.

### Dew claws

Many of those in favour of tail docking claim that the operation is done to prevent injury. Injuries to long tails are few and far between, however, when compared to torn dew claws (see page 122). They are often cut off at the same time as are the tails, with some exceptions such as the Pyrenean mountain dog, where fashion declares they be left on, supposedly to grip better when walking on snow.

### Ear cropping

Ear cropping is an illegal procedure in Australia and the United Kingdom. In countries where it is still practised, it is claimed that erect ears are less prone to infection than ones that hang down and that the dogs look smarter and much more fierce with their ears cropped. In a remote area in the Sierra Nevada in Spain, I witnessed the extraordinary double standard of seeing three Great Danes, with ears cropped for aesthetic effect, in a small village where there were many homeless, starving dogs unloved and uncared for by any owners. Where ear cropping is banned it is considered to be a mutilating operation.

### Debarking

This is illegal in most states in Australia, and is only carried out if a Statutory Declaration is made by the owner stating that the only other alternative is euthanasia. The dog can still bark, although it sounds as if it has a bad case of laryngitis.

Debarking is cruel in that it may disguise the fact that the owner is neglectful and unfeeling of the dog, leaving it bored, isolated and thus barking in the backyard. It also renders the dog ineffective as a guard!

The stressed barker yaps monotonously and regularly for hours on end or else barks at the slightest stimulus – cats, possums, passers-by harassing them; such behaviour also indicates extreme boredom. Some breeds bark more than others.

# 11

# Parasites

A parasite is a creature that lives in, on or off something without contributing anything in return, often to the detriment of the host. Sound familiar? Know anyone like that?

## INTERNAL PARASITES: WORMS

All worms cause some ill health in dogs. This is not surprising when you consider the nature of a parasite that lives off others and contributes nothing in return. A parasite obviously wants to go on living in a healthy host so it won't lose its free meal ticket but if that host gets run down, the mutual balance of parasite and host can get out of kilter and the worm ends up thriving at the expense of the host. The result: a very sick pup or dog.

### Roundworms
'Mummy! Mummy! Mitzi's done a pooh and it's got real live spaghetti in it. Yuk!' Poor little Ellie got a terrible shock when her family's new puppy, recently purchased from the markets, passed a whole pile of writhing roundworms. Her colourful description was in fact very apt. When she and her mother came to consult me, their first concern was whether Ellie could catch the worms. 'Should I worm the whole family?' asked Mrs Barlow.

'No,' I replied. 'Pups don't get threadworms from children and children cannot get this intestinal form of roundworms in their bowel. But they can be a health hazard to children in another way.' I went on to explain that mature roundworms in the pup's intestine lay eggs that pass out of the rectum and stick on the coat or contaminate the soil. After a while, depending on the amount of warmth and dampness in the area, the eggs become infective and, if accidentally swallowed by children, can migrate through the body and settle somewhere in the system as harmless little cysts. This condition, called *visceral larva migrans*, can be serious if the larvae settle somewhere like on the retina of the eye, causing disturbances to vision.

In the past this condition was hard to differentiate from a malignancy so that some children had an eye removed only to find it had not been necessary. Such cases were very rare but of course they made world media headlines. Now, more sophisticated scientific tests can be made to distinguish the two conditions and, of course, any risk can be eliminated by a proper worming programme for the dog.

'I suppose Ellie should wash her hands after she handles the pup,' said Mrs Barlow. 'Are you kidding?' I replied. 'I defy any mother to make their children religiously do that and, anyway, it takes all the spontaneity out of the pet–child relationship. Certainly it is wise to be careful after this first worming,' I said, popping some tablets down Mitzi's throat, 'and to pick up and dispose of the pup's droppings. But a correctly wormed pup is not a serious health hazard. You must give it worming syrup every week from 1 week of age until 6 weeks of age, then continue with tablets every fortnight until 3 months.' This treatment will stop the mature egg-laying adults from ever developing and therefore keep the environment from being contaminated. Failure to carry out a proper worming programme, however, can cause a real health hazard to toddlers crawling in long, lush grass.

Ellie had her nose all screwed up and she was standing well away from the surgery table with her hands behind her back. Poor Mitzi had suddenly taken on the appeal of a plague victim in Ellie's eyes. 'Come and give Mitzi a cuddle, Ellie. She needs you and she soon won't be carrying any more wiggly beasties in her,' I reassured the little girl. Ellie edged a little nearer to the table and held her pup. 'Right Ellie,' said her mother, 'off home now and wash your hands. Then I'll take you out to lunch for a holiday treat.' The last I heard Ellie say, as they left, was 'Mum, we're not going to the spaghetti place are we?'

You may wonder if it is safe to worm a bitch in pregnancy and if this will prevent the pups from getting roundworms. In fact, it is perfectly safe to worm a bitch in pregnancy and this precaution will prevent contamination of the environment as a future threat to the unborn pups. It will not, however, prevent the pups from being born with roundworm infestation because Nature has been most ingenious in perpetuating the life cycle of the roundworm. Even a regularly wormed bitch will have roundworm larvae encysted somewhere in her body. In some mysterious way, pregnancy mobilises these larvae to migrate to the puppies via the mother's bloodstream and placenta. The larvae can also contaminate the mother's milk. This is the reason it is essential to start a worming programme at about 1 week of age.

Apart from the human health hazard they present, heavy roundworm infestations can kill pups. As well as being infected from the dam, pups can easily get infected from their own droppings. The eggs go through a number of larval stages and then migrate through the liver and lungs where they are coughed up and swallowed into the stomach. Here, they grow into egg-laying adult worms again.

The sight of a heavily infested pup can tear at your heartstrings. It becomes pot-bellied with its skin stretched tight and the bones sticking out. It develops chronic diarrhoea, lacklustre eyes and may cough from lung damage due to the migrating larvae. This lung damage can also predispose it to pneumonia. Worms sometimes obstruct in a knot somewhere in the bowel and the larvae can inflame the ducts of the internal organs. Understandably, it looks depressed and cannot play like other pups. Be guided by your vet about the most up-to-date treatment of roundworms.

### Hookworm
The very name can cause your intestines to knot up at the thought of these creatures that attach to the bowel wall of a dog and suck blood. As in the case of roundworm, a pup can be born with hookworm, having been infected via the mother's bloodstream before birth or from the first milk. The same drugs that kill roundworm will work for hookworm so it is vitally important to worm a pup at regular intervals from about a week old. The syrup or tablets for pups covers both roundworm and hookworm and is given weekly from 1 week old to 6, then fortnightly to age 6 months.

Hookworm in dogs is not dangerous to humans. We have our own brand of hookworm, which occurs in hot, humid climates. Pups and humans can both get the infective larvae from soil penetrating the skin, usually of the feet, but in humans this stops at the cutaneous stage where the larvae cause red bumps that follow a little tract under the skin. These bumps then become itchy. This skin rash is known as *cutaneous larva migrans* or, more aptly, creeping eruption.

Pups are in great danger from hookworms, and they cannot be seen in a pup's droppings. Even examining a young pup's motion for worm eggs can fail to get results because the worms may not have reached the egg-laying stage even though they can already be causing serious symptoms. Hookworm loves a damp, hot, humid climate so pups in these areas are in danger. Those unfortunate pups who have not had a proper worming programme become anaemic and emaciated, get diarrhoea and can eventually die.

### Whipworm

Whipworms do not start to be a problem until the pup is over the roly-poly, puppy stage, so, up until the age of 3 months, worming for hookworm and roundworm is all that is necessary. At 3 months, usually when you are taking your dog to the vet for its shots, the worming programme for all types of worms can then begin. This worming should be repeated every 3 months. There are now pills that conveniently cover a dog for all types of hazardous intestinal worms.

Although not usually seen in the motions, whipworm can cause bad bouts of diarrhoea with mucus. The worms live in the caecum, a part of the bowel, and are caught by ingesting the infected larvae. Whipworm can live in soil for a long time so it can be very hard to eliminate the source of infection. As these worms also prefer a warm, humid climate, they are not found in every part of the world such as in the United Kingdom.

### Tapeworm

Dogs harbour many varieties of tapeworms and, as their name suggests, they are flattened like tape and composed of segments joined together. The front end of a tapeworm has a head. This is not your usual conception of a head, complete with eyes, nose, ears and a cute smile but a scolex with a rostellum that has hooks to hang onto the bowel wall. Nature is very precise in its design. The common town tapeworm, caught from fleas, has three or four rows of rosethorn-shaped hooks while one of its country-cousin worms has 44 large and small hooks arranged in two rows. Another fellow, caught from eating water creatures, has no hooks but a pair of elongated bothridia – no, its not in the *Oxford Pocket Dictionary* but I think it is best described as being like velcro.

As for the length this last creature grows to, it can reach 10 metres long in a dog or cat with as many as three thousand segments. This sounds formidable but the most dangerous tapeworm to health of humans is the country tapeworm *Echinococcus granulosus* causing hydatid disease, and it has only three or four segments.

Unlike the previous worms we have talked about, dogs are rarely really sick from tapeworms but to continue their life cycles the worms have to travel through an intermediate host that can itself become diseased as a result.

### *The common town tapeworm: Dipylidium caninum*

Mrs Carruthers was rather a snob. She loved impressing people, especially those high up the social scale. So one day she asked her new neighbour in for afternoon tea, probably served in bone china and accompanied by cucumber sandwiches and cake.

Mrs Carruthers told me her 'horror' story. While they were engaged in small talk, Mrs Carruthers's 6-month-old pup bounded into the room. 'My dear,' Mrs Carruthers recounted. 'There was Mrs Lanham-Jones, poised with a forkful of sponge cake at her open mouth, when in rushed Jessie, threw herself at the horrified woman's feet, tobogganed along on her bottom and left a writhing worm on the carpet! Imagine my embarrassment! Mrs Lanham-Jones will probably never speak to me again.' I had to quickly turn my back and fiddle with a row of pill pots to hide my laughter!

Jessie's social *faux-pas* was the result of an excruciating tickle caused by a tapeworm segment trying to wend its way out of the rectum. The worm in question was the common town variety. The ripe segments pass out of the anus looking like grains of rice or cucumber seeds. When you look closely at them you can see that they move like tiny concertinas, alternately long and then short, rather than just wiggling about like complete small worms of other varieties.

The dog catches tapeworm by eating a flea and not by direct contact with another dog. A flea larva eats a tapeworm egg, a dog then eats a flea and so the cycle of the tapeworm continues.

A well-cared-for young pup will probably not have tapeworms but if the dog is heavily infected with fleas, the chances are that it will become infected. On the market now are 'All-Wormers' that effectively dispatch all types of worms. Three-monthly administration of these tablets is adequate.

*The country tapeworm: Echinococcus granulosus*
There is a strange double standard that exists in homesteads in the Australian bush. A well-to-do property owner will have pampered pooches in the house, but the working dogs will be chained outside when not working and the owner will make no attempt to physically make a fuss of them. One of the reasons for this segregation is that there is a danger of the working dogs harbouring the small worm, composed of only a few segments, that carries the dreaded hydatid disease. This disease is caught by the dog eating raw, infected offal containing hydatid cysts that finally develop into a worm in the intestines. The eggs pass out of the dog with the faeces and can be picked up by man and domestic animals to grow into hydatid cysts somewhere in the body. The eggs can contain 'daughter' cysts inside and outside the egg, so many cysts can infect the host body.

The disease can take a heavy toll. An infected carcass has to be written off as an economic loss. A human may become fatally infected, mainly in the liver and lungs but sometimes in the brain, heart and bone.

New Zealand and Tasmania have to their credit a vigorous control programme. At a friend's deer farm in New Zealand I noticed that the dogs were kept kennelled on the day that the government dog-worming inspector called to personally administer the medicine. Yes, he still had 10 fingers! One of the dogs, Scott, a sheepdog who would normally not let a vet anywhere near him, wagged his tail with delighted anticipation when he knew the dosed meat was about to arrive.

The World Health Organisation has tackled the problem in South America but, in spite of government pamphlets distributed in country areas in Australia, it is still a significant problem here. Although this is sometimes blamed on migrant workers who cannot read English, there are many other surprising cases of ignorance. I actually witnessed an intelligent property-owner feed her working dogs raw offal, and considering how well known the danger of this disease is, I could not believe my eyes.

The problem is complicated by the fact that wild animals such as the dingo in Australia harbour the worm and the kangaroo, for example, can be an intermediate host, so it is virtually impossible to stamp out the disease in some areas.

If you live in the country, never feed raw offal from a carcass killed on the property. The offal should be incinerated; even boiling cannot guarantee to kill the cysts in a liver. Vegetable gardens should be kept enclosed so dogs cannot use them as a toilet. After handling working dogs, you should wash your hands. Dogs must be wormed with the appropriate medicine, as advised by your vet, every six weeks. Many dogs like to hang around abattoirs and this of course should be strictly policed.

What of the meat from your butcher? Although this has passed muster by the meat inspector, I still make it a precautionary rule to cut offal into small pieces and cook it thoroughly.

### Other country-cousins and foreign parasites

*Taenia hydatigena* is another country tapeworm but not harmful to humans. Its final host is the dog but as intermediate hosts it uses herbivores, whose livers become infected. *Taenia ovis*, found in the country dog, is the cause of 'sheep measles' where the intermediate stage of the worm encysts in the muscles of the meat and renders it unfit for human consumption.

*Spirometra erinacei* has an even fancier life cycle than most. As the tapeworm segments leave the dog they exist as a free-swimming organism that is eaten by such creatures as tiny crustaceans. These creatures in turn are swallowed by tadpoles, frogs and small rodents, by which stage the parasite has become a so-called sparganum. Man can also be a host. Dogs become infected by eating spargana-infected animals – not humans, hopefully!

Small pups can suffer from another kind of parasite called *Coccidium*, which often causes bad diarrhoea and is common in pups from markets and pounds. Dogs can also harbour *Giardia*, which may or may not cause symptoms of bad diarrhoea. People usually pick up this parasite when visiting the East but it has now become common in many other places, such as Australia, and can be caught from contaminated water.

Generally speaking the hotter the climate, the greater the parasite problem. Be advised by your vet concerning an efficient control programme as conditions vary from region to region and country to country. Such a programme can also vary according to the type of dog. Working and hunting dogs, for example, often need much more frequent worming than the well-heeled town pooch.

### Heartworm

Heartworm is on the increase worldwide and in the United States and Australia it has now spread to areas where it was never known before. The parasites are carried and transmitted by mosquitoes.

When an infected mosquito bites your dog, it injects larvae into the dog's system. These larvae undergo several bodily changes until the last stage when they migrate to the heart and settle in the heart chamber and coronary blood vessels. When they become mature adult worms, the females will begin to secrete hundreds of tiny larvae into the bloodstream, especially around dawn and dusk when the mosquitoes are biting. This process takes about five months.

Then when another mosquito bites your dog, it takes up the larvae with it and these undergo changes within the body of the mosquito for a period of 14–21 days until they become infective and are transferred to another dog by a mosquito bite, to begin the cycle all over again.

Dogs with the disease may show no symptoms while others tire easily and get a cough. If worms enter the right atrium of the heart, they cause the blood to churn up and the red cells become ruptured. As a result, the dog becomes severely distressed and passes red urine. If the dog is seen immediately by the vet, surgical removal of the worms from the heart is possible.

Dogs with heartworm get blocked blood vessels, which cause lack of blood supply to parts of the lungs. It does not take much imagination to understand how appallingly sick a dog must feel in the last stages of this disease before death. Treatment to kill the worms has its hazards, but a dog *can* be cured.

The disease is a terrible one, but it can so easily be avoided by the administration of heartworm preventative tablets. You have a choice of daily or monthly tablets. The former must be given every day without fail but are cheaper than the more convenient monthly tablets. All can be purchased in a palatable, chewable form if your dog is difficult to dose. One brand of tablets also eliminates intestinal worms (excluding tapeworm). Check with your vet if heartworm is in your area and commence the daily treatment at age 2 weeks and the monthly treatment at 6 weeks; it must be continued for life and not just during the mosquito season.

*Never* start a dog over 6 months of age on heartworm preventative tablets without a blood test first because, if there are larvae in the bloodstream, the dog can die of shock. A routine blood test will check that there are no larvae circulating in the blood. The dog might be suffering, however, from occult heartworm disease where there are only adult male worms present, in which case a normal filter test produces a negative result. Many vets now use an antigen test that also detects occult heartworm. If occult heartworm is suspected, there are other tests, such as radiology, ECG and other blood tests, to aid diagnosis.

# EXTERNAL PARASITES: FLEAS, TICKS, MANGE AND RINGWORM

## Fleas

These are 'great survivors, terrible guests'! One can only envy the flea – for its knees! Where would the world be without knees, essential to the likes of sportspersons, racehorses, chorus girls and even gangsters, known to gun their victims down at the knee. But the flea has the most remarkable pair in all Creation. Thanks to its incredible joints and a pad of super-elastic resin in the thorax, a flea can jump 150 times its own length with a blast-off capacity 50 times that of a space shuttle. And what's more, it doesn't get arthritis!

The flea is a super-survivor, thick-skinned in all senses of the word. Walk on one and it will hop away. Immerse one in water and it will come up spluttering. Fingernail-crushing is the only effective exterminator method if you manage to catch one red-handed. In the olden days, women wore flea-traps made of wood and ivory down the front of their bodice and they contained a blood-soaked rag to attract and catch the fleas.

Over the years the flea has become resistant to a whole range of insecticides so they are now even tougher customers. I wager that the flea, like the cockroach, will survive the bomb and inherit the earth! Carriers of the Great Plague via rats, fleas have been responsible throughout history for more deaths than both world wars and this death toll has not ended. Plague exists in some parts of the world even today.

There are more than 2400 species of flea and, although each type of animal has its own corresponding type of flea, fleas are not host-specific. This means in effect that dog fleas will go on cats and cat fleas on dogs and all of them will have a go at humans!

There are different types of flea such as sedentary fleas and stickfast fleas but the variety to concern pet owners is the hopping flea. These fleas are carriers of the common town tapeworm. Also some adults and often young children can be particularly allergic to bites from this type. They are thought strangely enough to be more attracted to women! Do we taste nicer?

There is still a definite social stigma attached to having fleas. Yet it is an inescapable fact of life, especially in warm, humid climates. Tell someone that their dog is scratching because it has fleas and it's on the cards that they will look you in the eye as if to say, 'Well, he must have caught them here at your place then!'

If your dog *is* scratching, it's worth checking its coat for fleas just in case. This is easier said than done because fleas are laterally depressed, which means they can shoot through a forest of dog-hairs at a mighty speed. Even if you are wearing strong reading-glasses, it can be hard to spot them, especially if your dog has a double coat.

A good trick to use to test for fleas is to ruffle the hair on the dog's back where the fleas will then beat a hasty retreat to the underside of the dog. Then, if you roll the dog over, the fleas should be caught out in the open, running across the bare tummy.

Young pups are particularly at risk from fleas as they can die from flea anaemia. Fleas eat blood. Later in life, pups can develop an allergy to the saliva of its fleas and this can sometimes linger for weeks after the last flea has bitten the dust.

## A flea's life cycle

The tiny fleas on your pup are males and the big, fat ones are females, full of eggs. The eggs are laid in the general environment but also on the animal and they look like tiny grains of salt, easily visible to the naked eye. Flea eggs unfortunately are resistant to insecticides.

The fleas hatch out into larvae, like tiny fly maggots, which feed on dirt and become tiny pupae or cocoons. At this stage they lie dormant in floor cracks, carpets and dog's bedding for months, until weather conditions are favourable for hatching a new generation of fleas.

The whole life cycle of the flea can be a matter of days in damp, warm weather or it can take months and months if conditions are not right. Have you ever walked into your house after a holiday when the place has lain empty – to suddenly find an infestation of fleas? The vibrations of your feet can be enough to hatch the pupae into a new generation of adult fleas, which immediately leap onto your legs for a feed! Even when deprived of an instant feast, unfed adult fleas can live for some months also.

*Dealing with fleas: the choices*
When dogs who are obviously suffering from flea allergy are brought to my surgery, a high percentage of owners tell me that they deflea their dog every night and catch about twenty fleas in a comb. I usually then say, 'But it is impossible to catch every flea on your dog and it takes only one to cause an allergy!'

They still do not believe me. A pet simply acts as a vacuum cleaner for all the fleas in the environment. Kill a flea on the animal, and there are plenty more to take its place.

It seems obvious to me then that, unless you tackle the dog's surroundings, treating the dog for fleas is pointless. You are just subjecting it to a bombardment of insecticides which, in the long term, are bound to have serious side effects; many insecticides, for example, are linked to cancer.

Some years ago fleas were not really a problem because chlorinated hydrocarbons, such as DDT and Dieldrin, were being used as powders and rinses. These had a residual effect, however, and hung about in the environment for years and years, building up to dangerous levels that contaminated the soil and consequently the vegetation and the animals feeding upon it. Although these flea rinses may have lasted a long time as flea deterrents, the environment and probably the pets themselves suffered as a result. These products are now thankfully banned. Most flea controls, in the form of flea rinses and collars, contain organophosphates and carbamate these days, but even some of these can be toxic.

## Tackling the dog
*Flea collars*
Most flea collars exude tiny particles of insecticide spray or liquid that spread through the animal's coat. Some pets are allergic to flea collars and develop a rash around the neck. Medallions or collars with the insecticide enclosed prevent contact with the skin and thus avoid this problem. I personally do not like flea collars because we do not really know what effect inhaling insecticide long-term can have on a dog. Nor do we have any way of knowing how the animal feels if, for example, it has a terrible headache.

Some owners have reported mood changes in their pets but at this stage these reports are purely circumstantial evidence that no one has properly researched. There are too many unanswered questions. Whatever the case may be, pets should not wear flea collars where there are any small children, who can easily handle or chew them with unhealthy results.

Manufacturers claim that the insecticide in flea collars is not absorbed by the pet but acts directly on the flea and that the minimal amount of insecticide absorbed into the system is nothing compared to a weekly flea rinse. If you *are* sold on flea collars, however, a small pup should not wear one until it has grown considerably. If your dog is a small breed it is also better for it to wear a cat flea collar. Always remove a new collar from packaging and air for 24 hours before putting it on your dog.

Never double up on insecticides by using another form of flea control such as an insecticidal rinse at the same time. Also beware of two pups wearing flea collars playing together as they can swing on each other's collars and get a dose of insecticide orally.

### Flea rinses and shampoos

Many shampoos incorporate an insecticide so the dog can be cleaned and defleaed at the same time. If the dog is already clean (overbathing should be avoided as it washes out the coat's natural oils), then you can use a flea rinse on its own. Brush the animal first and then apply the rinse. Owners have a bad habit of not reading instructions carefully. They often apply the rinse at the wrong strength, slinging an unmeasured quantity in a bucket. 'No worries,' they think until the animal gets sick. Some people, for example, complain to me, 'But we've rinsed him *every* day to keep the fleas off', when the instructions clearly stated that only weekly rinses were necessary.

The safest insecticide to use on puppies is natural pyrethrum, which can be obtained in the form of powder, shampoo or spray, and is perfectly safe where there are young children handling dogs. (Some of these sprays contain the insect growth hormone inhibitor which stops fleas breeding on the dog.) Pyrethrum comes from a type of chrysanthemum but, as there are not enough flowers available to meet the demand, synthetic pyrethrums are on the market that are just as safe. Your vet will advise you of the brand names in your particular part of the world.

Remember when out shopping for anti-flea rinses or shampoos that ingredients of products should be written on the packet, even if they are nearly always in very small print.

### Ultrasonic collars

These emit a high-frequency sound, inaudible to the human ear but which fleas cannot stand. They do not in fact kill fleas but are reputed to help keep them away from the animal. Many have proved useless, but models developed in the United States are reasonably effective.

### Oral insecticides

These are organophosphates that are fed as drops or tablets and act systemically, that is to say through the whole body, to kill fleas. We do not at this stage know how this makes the animal feel nor what are the long-term effects of this treatment.

## *Other insecticidal treatments*
There are on sale to the general public small tubes containing organophosphate insecticides that are squeezed onto the animal behind the neck. In about eight hours this is absorbed into the fat deposits of the body from where it acts against the fleas without actually circulating through the entire body's system. Applying this treatment to the dog last thing at night eliminates the risk of children and adults accidently touching the area where the insecticide is being absorbed and therefore getting contaminated on the hands and mouth. This treatment takes about three days to have effect and must be repeated at regular intervals according to the instructions. It is not to be used on small puppies, so follow the directions carefully. Also be vigilant as skin allergy around the neck is possible in some dogs.

## Tackling the environment
### *Vacuuming*
This helps enormously in flea control. Put some flea powder in the vacuum bag first and then empty the bag afterwards, onto newspaper away from the house. Incinerate if possible.

The food that larvae feed on as well as flea eggs and some fleas will be vacuumed up but not all of them of course, particularly as larvae have hooks that tend to hang onto carpets. Unfortunately, flea plagues always seem to occur in the hottest weather, which is when you least feel like vacuuming!

### *Clean bedding*
Wash the dog's bedding regularly in hot, soapy water and hang it outside in sunlight to dry. Rinsing the bedding in the dog's flea rinse can also be useful.

### *Sprays*
The only really safe household spray is one containing pyrethrum or its synthetic equivalent. This has a knockdown effect on the fleas, stunning them for a while. Some may recover, so vacuum the area and dispose of the cleaner's contents after spraying to get rid of as many fleas as possible.

### *Insect growth hormone inhibitors*
These are the biggest breakthrough ever in flea control. The active ingredient is the same as that used in malarial control to kill the mosquito larvae in drinking water and has been passed by the World

Health Organisation. This fact alone gives one some degree of confidence that it is safe to administer where there are pets and humans.

The flea larvae hatch out of the eggs and then do not survive, so it virtually acts as a birth control mechanism for fleas. It is used in the form of a mist spray so you must close up the house and vacate it for two hours. The effect lasts for about seven months. You should also soak the garden with water at the same time so larvae outside cannot survive and put a flea shampoo on the dog to kill the existing population of fleas. Hosing garages and outside concrete areas will thoroughly finish the job.

The mist-spray pack can be obtained from vets and other outlets. The effectiveness of this treatment can be diminished if the areas sprayed are usually washed with alkaline detergent, so it is recommended that you vacuum wooden floors instead of washing them. The product works particularly well where there are carpets.

There is also an oral insect growth hormone inhibitor, which is given monthly, that stops fleas breeding on a dog.

*Alternative flea control: biosphere-friendly products*
With the ever-increasing number of people becoming aware of the many threats to our environment from the poisons we pour into it, it is no wonder that there is concern about the long-term effects of many of the insecticides we use on ourselves and our pets. Apart from their toxic hazards, insecticides can contain ingredients to which dogs are allergic.

A great deal of scientific research has been done on the possible harmful effects of insecticides. For example, in experiments dogs have been fed the substances that are put in flea collars with no apparent ill-effects. In West Germany, concern was expressed about the dangers to children from touching flea collars containing *carbaryl*. It was claimed, after tests, that the amount that children would absorb was well below the recommended level for safety.

Such scientific claims still pose the question whether there is any safe level long-term. Although currently approved insecticides are eliminated fairly rapidly from the body, what does a regular toxic shock in small doses ultimately do to the body's system? This has not been adequately answered. If you have any doubts, there are many natural products now available that have been used by many people with great success. As a columnist about pets for many years, I have quite a collection of readers' remedies that they swear by. Be aware that some natural products also can cause an allergic reaction.

*Flea collars* mostly contain pyrethrum, pennyroyal or herbal oils that repel insects.

*Shampoos* Pennyroyal and other flea and insect-repelling herbs.

*Flea powders*   often contain aromatic herbs such as pennyroyal, eucalyptus, citronella, rosemary, rue and wormwood.

*Lemon skin tonic*   helps keep fleas away and is made by cutting up
a lemon, putting in a pint of almost boiling water and leaving overnight.
It can be sponged onto the dog's coat and allowed to dry. It also helps
with the irritating skin problems associated with fleas.

*Methylated spirit*   sprayed on the fleas seems to kill them, but could
be drying to the skin.

*Wash your dog in oatmeal soap*   and then apply tea-tree oil, rubbing
it into the affected areas. Too much tea-tree oil, or using it on raw areas,
can be dangerous.

*Fennel seeds*   Boil them up and then use this infusion to wash floors
as a flea-deterrent.

*Brewer's yeast*   sprinkled on the food and also rubbed in the coat,
helps many dogs combat the effect of fleas.

*Eucalyptus oil*   dabbed on the dog, acts as a flea-deterrent but do not
overuse it.

*Crushed garlic*   in food also seems to deter fleas.

### The intense flea-sufferer

Dogs vary in their tolerance to fleas. Some dogs overreact to the presence
of a single flea by scratching until they have a weeping, red, pus-covered
sore while other dogs, whose immune systems are good, may have quite
a few fleas galloping over them but do not appear to react at all.

If you have a panting, scratching, highly distressed dog whose whole
life is made an absolute misery by fleas, then you should seriously
consider the sensible use of insecticides. Otherwise, the dog's life will
not be worth living. If there is no alternative to using insecticides for
a severe flea-sufferer, try to take a break from flea control in the winter
months when there are no fleas around. This break will cleanse out
the dog's system.

### Ticks: potential killers

One day a rather slurred voice came on the telephone. 'She's chicks all
over, come quick, can't get 'em off.' The phone tumbled to the floor with
a clatter. I hoped the caller hadn't followed it because I did not have a
clue as to the address. The voice eventually came back and I was given
a vague street name and number. When I got there, I found a nervous
cocker spaniel who showed no signs of tick poisoning at all, and a
drunken owner who had been trying to pull a harmless wart off her dog!
Even people who are not in their cups can be misled about the
appearance of a tick. Small growths, warts and scabs are all at some time
mistaken for ticks.

## A tick's life cycle and distribution

The tick, *Ixodes holocyclus*, is only present along the eastern scrub-areas of Australia where the natural host is native wildlife who are immune to its poison. It is, however, a potential killer of pets. Dogs and cats become accidental hosts and can die a horrible death.

The life cycle of the tick is in three stages. In the first stage, it is often called a grass or seed tick and is smaller than a pinhead, somewhat resembling a minute spider. Although not really poisonous, it sucks blood and some people can have a sensitive reaction to its bites. Ticks in the second stage are also pretty harmless and, rejoicing in the name of 'nymphs', they reach a length of 3 mm after gorging on blood.

Stage number three is the killer! Only the adult female is poisonous and not the male. She sucks the blood from four days up to a week when symptoms in the host start to develop. Fully engorged, she can be up to 13 mm long with a smooth, greyish appearance, like a shiny sac.

## Getting it off

People often panic and rush for a bottle of kerosene as soon as they spot a tick on their dog. They then pour it on the animal and wonder why it develops a bad burn!

The fascinating thing about the tick is that she cannot detach herself until she has injected a type of enzyme that digests the skin area into which she is embedded. Only then can she drop off.

So to dislodge her, you have to take her by surprise and engage in quite a duel of strength. Raise the dog's skin between thumb and fore-finger and, with tweezers level with the skin, give a quick jerk sideways. She should then come off with quite a snap.

People often panic because they think they have left the head behind. Squashing the body of the tick with your fingers while trying to pull it out could, I guess, get it mad and stimulate it to shoot some poison in at a furious rate, so vets often inject a little of the dose of anti-tick serum under the skin where the tick was embedded. By getting the tick out with tweezers, the head usually comes away and if you look closely you can even see it. Leaving the head behind is in fact no big deal as no more poison will enter the dog as a result and the dog will at worst get just a rough, infected sore.

## Symptoms

An observant owner rang me one day to report that his male dog's voice had gone up several octaves, making him a suitable candidate for the King's College Choir, Cambridge. The dog's bark had indeed gone high-pitched and this is one of the very first symptoms of tick poisoning.

The dog may occasionally vomit and then a stagger appears in the back legs. This stagger gradually moves to the front part of the body until the dog is unable to stand and develops laboured, rasping breathing and dry retching. When this happens, the respiratory muscles have been paralysed and the end is near.

A small percentage of dogs will make a spontaneous recovery in mild cases, which accounts for the reputed success of so many 'old wives' tales' treatments with no basis in scientific proof.

Tick serum, although expensive, is invaluable in saving a dog's life. When the dog has a serious case of tick poisoning, it needs to be hospitalised so it can have supportive treatment such as fluids injected to feed it and drugs to control the vomiting and other symptoms.

A dog with tick poisoning should be kept very quiet after its recovery and should not be allowed to bake in the hot sun. Some dogs can become immune to tick poisoning but many do not. Because you have successfully removed one tick, do not assume that there will not be another hidden in the coat. Shaggy dogs often need clipping when they display early symptoms of poisoning and you have been unable to locate a tick.

*Prevention*
No preventative measure can replace the daily search for ticks, especially if you live in a tick area. Although mostly picked up around the head, ticks can be found anywhere on a dog, so do not leave a hair unturned! Make your inspection thorough: look around the anus, in the mouth and ears, up the nose and between the toes. Feeling for ticks through the coat is generally more effective than actually looking for them.

The use of insecticidal soaps and rinses weekly will help to prevent poisoning, as can internal insecticides. Specific collars to deter ticks are also available. But do not depend totally on these methods.

Clipping long-coated dogs in hot weather makes routine searching easier and of course makes the dog a lot more comfortable anyway.

**Mange**
*Demodectic mange: the moth-eaten look*
'My pup looks all moth-eaten on the feet and a bit on the head!' said Mr Parsons. 'It does not seem to worry him at all but it is not getting any better and seems to be spreading.' Some skin scrapings, examined under the microscope, showed it to be the mange mite, prevalent in young dogs under 1 year old. They acquire the mite from the mother when she is suckling, which is why it is usually distributed around the head and feet.

The mites look like tiny cigars that have settled in the hair follicles. This form of the mite can disappear spontaneously and is often carried in dogs who never show any symptoms whatsoever.

There is another form, however, that can become generalised and occurs in dogs of all ages. Secondary bacterial infection sets in very quickly in these cases and can sometimes become impossible to treat successfully. One can assume that there is something very wrong with the dog's immune system if this happens. Treatment is with drugs that are highly toxic if not used correctly, so listen to and read your vet's instructions very carefully when you carry out the treatment.

### Sarcoptic mange or scabies: the scurfy look

This usually occurs in older dogs but if pups get it, they usually get it all over their body. The condition is very itchy with red lumps and crusts and sometimes there is a generalised scurfy or scaly look.

Scabies in people was very common in the olden days and very much associated with poverty and dirty surroundings but it can pop up here and there in the most unlikely places. It is the sort of condition that, if you and your dog get it, you are likely to keep quiet about, or you will be struck off your friends' visiting lists! Insecticidal rinses are usually effective.

### Ringworm

Ringworm is a highly deceptive name for this condition. It's not a worm chasing its own tail but a fungus that attacks the hair follicles, making them fall out and then spreading in an ever-increasing circle to form a scaly round patch, usually around the head and feet. People can be very emotional about pets with ringworm. One woman rushed in to my surgery with her pup held at arm's length, demanding its demise. 'Why, we might catch it!' she shrieked.

'It's hardly life-threatening if you do,' I said. 'I made it a great excuse to stay away from school once when I caught it off a calf but it isn't the end of the world.' I told her to get checked by the doctor; if he so advised, the family could get tablets to stop it breaking out in them while the pup was being treated. When a pet has a skin disease infectious to humans, one immediately tends to start scratching, and to feel nervous about laying your head on a cushion lest it be covered in infected hair and you end up having to shave your head and look like a skinhead! With baths, lotions and creams, tablets taken internally, and attention to hygiene, your pup can be cured. It's certainly not ready for the big jump!

Offputting though this chapter may sound to the potential dog owner, if you take simple preventative measures, nothing need be a danger to you and yours. You risk much more on a crowded bus!

PART IV

# Some Big Issues Tackled

# 12

# Your Dog and the Law: Insurance

## 'I'LL SEE YOUR DOG IN COURT'

Dog insurance? Well, to be honest, I wasn't thinking along the lines of you taking out a life policy on your pet so that when he met with a sudden demise you would be compensated for the emotional loss with enough money for a world trip! No such policies exist in Australia, anyway, and no amount of money could ever compensate for such a loss. But I do urge all new dog owners to take out a policy that will insure themselves against any damage that their dog may do to persons or property. 'But,' I hear you object immediately, 'I have a sweet-natured dog who, raised and cared for according to the guidelines of this book, is not capable of harming a fly. So why do I need insurance?' Famous last words. Some very bizarre and totally unexpected incidents can occur.

Cashew, a lively crossbreed of my acquaintance, was given as a present to a grandmother. She loved him dearly but he was the wrong sort of dog for her because of his hyperactive nature. I was walking through the park one day with a friend of mine, who is of rather generous proportions, when we bumped into Cashew and his elderly owner. Cashew, coming full-pelt in the other direction, bumped into my large friend and caught her at the back of the knees. She was felled like a bowling pin. Luckily for Cashew's owner, my friend did not sue for damages that would have included weeks off work with a broken foot. 'Cashew did not mean to do it,' was all she said.

Some owners are not so lucky in this age of sue and be sued. There

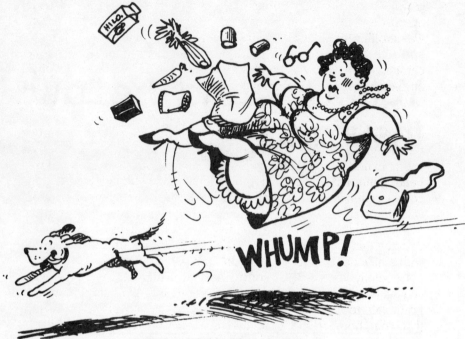

*Cashew felled her like a ninepin.*

was, for example, the case of a German shepherd dog named Carmen who at age 13 was going deaf. One hot summer's day she was asleep in the driver's seat of her owner's car with the car window wound half-down to give her some air. A parking cop bent down to chalk-mark the front wheel and his broad shoulder slightly protruded through the open window. Carmen woke in fright and nipped the parking cop on the shoulder.

The bruise on the cop's shoulder did not even break the skin but the case ended up in court. Due to excellent references from vets, dog trainers and personal friends, corroborated by displays of photos showing Carmen being hugged tightly by a bunch of handicapped children, this German shepherd dog got off with, in the judge's words, 'an unblemished character'. Though Carmen's life was spared, the owner had to pay quite a hefty sum to the cop for the inconvenience of the tiny bruise, and a new shirt.

And what of the case of the young Rhodesian ridgeback who slipped out the front gate right into heavy peak-hour traffic and ran straight into a car? The dog sustained an uncomplicated leg fracture that healed completely but you should have seen the terrible state of the Mercedes Benz! Luckily the dog owner was adequately insured.

Then there's the case of Bounce the Boxer, well named for his boisterous nature. In a quiet street in the mountains, Bounce in his usual manner decided to plant an enthusiastic kiss on an old pensioner who was strolling the sidewalk. Bounce's clumsy knock against the old man's arm with its delicate, paper-thin skin caused a nasty sore that later became infected. This was another case that ended in court and involved an animal of good temperament whose intentions were anything but savage.

I maintain that there is potential for biting lurking in every dog no matter how seemingly sweet natured it may be. A sudden scare can be enough to cause a fear–bite reaction. In one case I heard about, a young child let out a blood-curdling scream as if Dracula himself was bearing him off just at the moment that a big dog bounded around the corner. Naturally the dog was startled. A small nip on the boy's bottom was the only result but the child's father claimed that his son had recurring nightmares of the incident and had suffered psychological damage that would mar him for life. All because a middle-aged dog with a nice nature and clean record had bitten out of fright.

Hopefully you are now convinced that taking out insurance is essential. Policies vary from company to company. Also, liability laws vary from state to state in Australia and in other countries. So make sure that your household public liability policy covers you should, for example, your dog bite the mail deliverer while on your premises. See to it that you are covered by a personal legal liability clause as an extension of your household policy for any accidents that occur off your premises. If you are travelling interstate or to another country, make sure you are still properly covered by your policy.

# IDENTIFICATION: DOG TAGS AND MICROCHIPS

A chapter on the legal status of dogs would not be complete without some comment on identification. Put a collar and dog-tag on your puppy from the moment that you get it. There is always someone who carelessly leaves a gate open. Young dogs are notorious for lacking road sense and pedigree pups make tempting prizes for thieves. Either way you don't want to lose your new pup by not having him properly labelled so that a kind neighbour or passerby can bring him home.

In this age of microtechnology it is possible to have a microchip, no bigger than the end of a matchstick, inserted under the dog's ear under local anaesthetic so that the dog has a permanent ID number. I am sure the average dog would not object to this practice on the grounds of invasion of privacy!

Dogs who end up in pounds but who were wearing collars when they got lost are often found without a collar. This obviously means someone had deliberately removed the dog's collar. On a tour of a dog museum in Leeds Castle in England, I saw what seemed to me the ideal solution – a mediaeval, brass, hinged collar with a key to lock it on. I only hope that the dog-owning knights of old were more careful with their dog-collar (and chastity-belt) keys than I am with my car keys!

## Registration

In Australia dogs must be registered with the local council. This entails a fee, which varies from state to state. There are discounts for pensioners and owners of dogs that have been desexed.

# 13

# Desex or Not Desex?: A Difficult Question

## DESEXING THE FEMALE: SOME QUESTIONS ANSWERED

Mrs Williams was holding her 3-month-old schnauzer, Isolde, on the surgery table for her vaccinations. 'Do you think that Isolde should have a litter before she is desexed?' she asked. 'Most people say they should.'

'Yes,' I said, 'but ask them "why" and you'll find that they are judging the situation in terms of human beings. Isolde is a much-loved family member but she is a dog after all and not a person. So of course she reacts differently. She won't know what she's missed if she doesn't have a litter and she won't bemoan her deprived state with her friends or drool over the pram of someone else's baby!'

'When you put it like that, I'm having second thoughts,' replied Mrs Williams, 'but I thought it might be educational for the children to see her have pups.'

'You're right there,' I said. 'Also, Isolde is a registered bitch from a popular breed so you wouldn't have much trouble selling the pups. But I warn you that an enormous amount of work is involved in arranging a suitable mating, and in rearing the pups correctly.'

'No, I'm not being realistic,' Mrs Williams reconsidered. 'We really have not the time to take this on properly. I think I'll opt for desexing after all. How old should she be?'

'The best time is when she is about 6 months old because the operation is simplest and cheapest then.' I went on to say that I favoured waiting until about three months after the first season – bitches come on heat twice a year for three weeks, usually from about 8 months old. This means they will be more developed physically and tend to put on less weight after the operation. They also somehow retain more feminine charm at that age – in fact, some bitches can be downright flirty! But you will have to be prepared for the queue of canine suitors gathered in your street during that first season. Don't forget either that these eager dogs can scale 2-metre fences and ardent bitches have been known to dig their way out underneath a fence. That all lasts three weeks, with the dangerous week in the middle when they will accept the male.

The first signs of a bitch being in season are a swollen vulva and a blood discharge. This can be copious in some bitches and make quite a mess. Up-market pet shops even sell special pants for 'that difficult time of the month'. After a few days, the bleeding stops and the discharge clears to a mucus type. Bitches will accept a male sometimes between the tenth and fourteenth day, although there can be some variation. Everything tails off during the third week despite some persistent male dogs still hanging around.

'Sounds like fun!' said Mrs Williams after hearing all this. 'I think we can happily give that a miss and we'll book her in when she's 7 months old or so,' decided Mrs Williams, 'but there is something else that

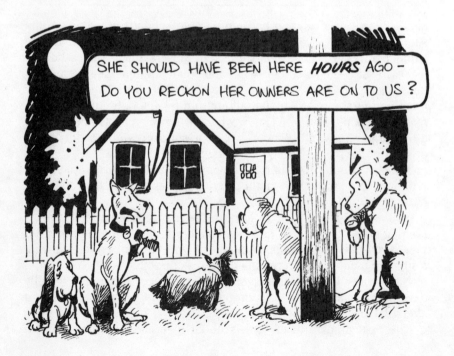

worries me. Wouldn't she develop osteoporosis if she is too young? My mother has this and I wouldn't wish it on a dog!'

'Good question,' I said, 'but we don't seem to find this problem in desexed bitches. I am convinced that this is because dogs don't smoke or drink alcohol and are usually on a balanced diet and take plenty of exercise!' The condition of post-menopausal calcium depletion in women, with the resulting 'dowager's hump' and crumbling bones that are easily prone to fractures, is indeed a terrible affliction of the elderly.

Mrs Williams still seemed doubtful about the idea of desexing. 'Now, there must be some minuses as well as pluses in this desexing business. What are they?' she queried.

'Well, there is a slight tendency to put on weight,' I explained, 'but this is easily kept in check by not overfeeding and by giving adequate exercise. Also, some bitches develop incontinence due to a hormone deficiency later in life. They can then involuntarily dribble small amounts of urine where they lie, as well as being smelly. A bitch gets upset about this but the condition is easily and cheaply controlled by hormone replacement therapy in tablet form.'

'Does it change a bitch's personality to be desexed?' Mrs Williams asked.

'No, not at all,' I replied. 'It's a common misconception that personality depends totally on sexuality! A bitch's personality remains basically the same, except that it is perhaps on a more even keel, without the manic swings of mood with which the human female is so familiar.' Mrs Williams finally went off, happy with her decision about Isolde. But what of the people whose prejudices cannot be broken down regarding desexing? What problems are they going to face with a lifetime of living with an undesexed bitch?

**Life with an undesexed bitch**
First, they have to contend with the six-monthly seasons. The dogged determination of some canine casanovas knows no bounds so don't mistakenly think it is safe to leave a bitch locked up in a yard. Even locking her in the house, carrying her to a car at night to drive to a far distant park and then exercising her on a leash so she does not make a bolt for it, will not stop attentive male dogs from picking up a wind scent and hanging around outside your premises. Here, their sexual rivalry gets them into serious dog fights on your doorstep!

The pack situation that then develops can become a public menace and a danger, particularly to small children. A dog in a pack behaves quite differently to how he would as an individual, the way some people behave in a rowdy football crowd. It is, of course, illegal to have a bitch on the street while she is in season and by nights all other dogs should be under the control of their owners. In practice of course this just does not happen.

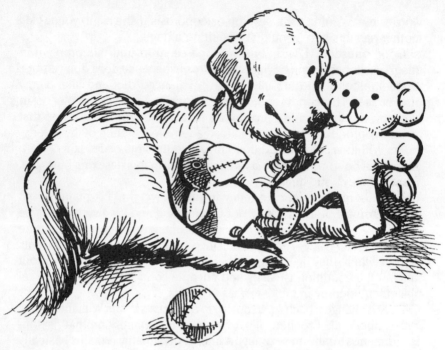

*False pregnancy in the undesexed bitch.*

The bitch in season can have serious fights with other bitches, being more moody at this time, even when she is not normally a fighter and would usually put other dogs, who are annoying her or pestering her pups, in their place with a warning snarl.

About six weeks after they have been in season, bitches often get a false pregnancy. This involves swelling in the abdomen and becoming very 'sooky' with behaviour such as taking children's cuddly toys into cupboards to nurse as imaginary pups. They even sometimes produce milk and many an owner is thereby totally convinced their bitch was 'got at' without their knowing. This bout of 'motherhood' passes off by itself without treatment but the 'mother' should not be given milk to drink during this time and should have plenty of exercise to take her mind off her imagined condition.

A bitch who is not desexed before the age of 2 years develops a high risk of mammary cancer. Owners should be aware of this and carry out regular check-ups. Any suspicious lumps should be examined by the vet.

From middle to old age, the undesexed bitch can also develop pyometra, a type of uterus infection probably brought on by hormone imbalance. If suffering from pyometra, the bitch is usually swollen in the abdomen, may drink and urinate excessively and exude a sticky, brown-reddish discharge from the vagina. In a so-called 'closed case', where the cervix is not open, there is no sign of discharge and the abdomen swells even more. Pyometra is an emergency. At the slightest sign of symptoms, see the vet straight away for a confirmation of diagnosis as immediate surgery is needed. Neglect of these cases leads to death. Treating with antibiotics and hormones is not effective. The risk of this operation is much greater than the risk of having a bitch desexed earlier in life, when any risks are almost nil.

The canine contraceptive pill, as an alternative to desexing, is not justifiable. It emulates pregnancy and the bitch becomes overweight and may develop serious side effects. Desexing the bitch is a must for the responsible dog owner. Every year there is a canine holocaust when thousands of dogs are put down on account of the appalling stray population problem.

# DESEXING THE MALE: MALE AGGRESSION AND EGO

Desexing a male dog is a much more controversial issue because there isn't the possibility of giving birth to pups to sway the decision one way or the other. Male owners tend to be against desexing as they usually take the issue personally. The issue of sexuality rates highly in the mind of the average human male.

Generally speaking, there is not such a strong case for desexing the male dog as there is for the female. His sexual urges may be easily contained by the owner, compared for example with the problems of restraining a tomcat, who will roam far and wide and sire hundreds of kittens, adding more numbers to the already large population of stray cats.

It is true that, after desexing, male dogs do tend to put on more weight than females. Often their bones do not take the weight increase too well and this can result in early arthritis. Some dogs, however, are far better off desexed.

Take the case of Miss Harmon and her silkie. From the time when he was a tiny pup, she protected him with all the motherly instincts that she had been unable to bestow upon a human child. Miss Harmon was elderly and frail and when she went to the park with Pixie she snatched him to her bosom and waved a stick if she saw a large dog approaching.

So it was not surprising when she came to the surgery one day with Pixie pouring blood from a wound on the back leg, where a male dog had attacked him, defenceless in his owner's arms. 'I always have him on a lead (poor Pixie!) and I picked him up when I saw the dog. Pixie barked so bravely but the dog attacked!' the distraught Miss Harmon sobbed.

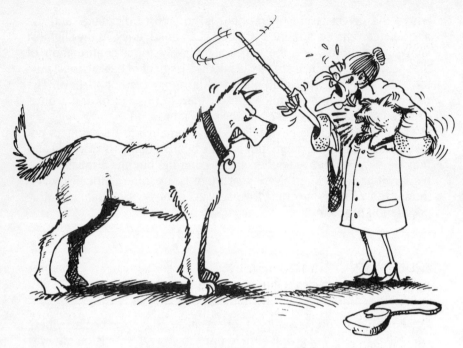

*Owners often unwittingly cause dog fights.*

What Miss Harmon did not realise was that she had instigated the whole incident by bringing up Pixie the wrong way. Small breeds of dogs have more than their fair share of male hormones in relation to their size and most have a very highly developed male ego to go with it. They walk with a positive swagger and arrogantly cock their leg so high when marking territory or just urinating that they nearly topple over. Small dogs are therefore not naturally timid or defenceless for their size and can handle 'social' situations with other dogs perfectly well.

If two unleashed male dogs are allowed to meet in a park, they will usually sort out who is top dog without any serious confrontation. Their owners, who are often elderly, do not realise this and their fear of the situation is transmitted to their dog, which then reinforces its show of fear–aggression, especially when the dog is restrained. This reaction then incites the other dog to become more aggressive and even to attack.

If Pixie had been allowed to meet other dogs from when he was a puppy, he would have developed, under natural circumstances and off the leash in a park, normal doggy relationships and minimised the chances of being attacked.

*Large* aggressive dogs can be very hard to handle. As I warned in Chapter 2 (page 12), if such a dog has been allowed to urinate on almost every upright post in his street when going for walks on a leash, he will develop a very strong territorial feeling about his area. As a result, battle royals may well become the status quo between a couple of neighbour's dogs every time they meet. Heeling your dog firmly until you reach the park will curb his feeling of owning the street exclusively.

If, however, you have ended up with an incurably aggressive male dog, desexing may well help the situation. Most aggression is usually but not inevitably sex-linked. In cases where it is sex-related, desexing is usually carried out in conjunction with behavioural drugs.

# SOME FALLACIES AND FACTS OF LIFE: LOVE AND SEX

One of the worst arguments for desexing a male dog is that an owner believes that it 'will quieten him down'. A dog has a great deal of natural exuberance until it has matured, which is not until it is 2 years of age in the larger breeds. A truly hyperactive dog is born that way because of its genetic make-up or it has been made that way, often because children have overstimulated it as a pup by playing with it in an uncontrolled way.

There are dogs, however, who are genuinely oversexed. These dogs, both large and small, will remain oversexed all their lives and, as there is no equivalent of a brothel for dogs, there are not outlets for their sexual frustration. Dogs such as these are better off desexed, because they can become an incredible nuisance with people and are unhappy in themselves. Not content with humping cushions, they will jump on people's legs if they are small dogs while larger ones can jump on children and sometimes become quite aggressive in their excitement.

Then there are the lovesick male dogs. Some highly strung, big, nervous dogs, who have become particularly strongly bonded to a female owner and have not been properly conditioned to accepting other dogs as their own kind, can literally fall in love with their owners. This can lead to all sorts of embarrassment.

One client exclaimed in despair, 'Why on earth is he doing that?' when her dog, gazing raptly at its owner, proceeded to have an erection. 'Because he is in love with you!' I explained. The poor woman did not know where to look. Her life and that of the dog were much more comfortable after the dog was desexed.

There are, however, some situations where you had hoped that a dog's behaviour would improve with desexing but it doesn't turn out to be a total success.

Roberta Jansen was a designer who mainly worked at home, so her 5-year-old Maltese male dog, a toy breed of considerable charm, was constantly with her and, not surprisingly, became very bonded to her. Unfortunately, he also came to loathe other dogs. Roberta finally met a young man with whom she began a steady relationship and they decided to live together. The dog had other ideas.

Roberta came to me about the problem. 'He hates my boyfriend,' she said, 'and tries to stop him coming near me. He even tries to bite him. If we lock him out of the bedroom, he howls and tears the place apart.'

'That's a typical stress reaction to separation from the owner,' I said, 'and he is jealous too – one human characteristic we can confidently attribute to dogs.'

'What can we do?' Roberta pleaded. 'I adore that dog but I don't want to spend the rest of my life married to him! I need a man more than a dog!'

'How does your boyfriend feel about dogs generally?' I asked.

'He likes them,' she said. 'And funnily enough he likes Joe. I can't think why!'

'Get him to take Joe out for walks and always feed him,' I advised. 'This may help.' Finally we decided to desex Joe and the situation did improve greatly but it was not completely solved as Joe's behaviour was so well entrenched after many years. Nonetheless, I'm happy to report that Roberta still has her boyfriend!

A male dog can be desexed at any age but should not be done under 1 year of age. Many young dogs go through an irritating adolescent stage when they make a nuisance of themselves but later this wears off, so desexing should not be performed in haste.

Middle-aged and older dogs should always have their testicles checked. If they feel enlarged or lumpy, this is a sure sign of cancer of the testicles, which requires immediate castration. Enlarged prostate glands in dogs cause difficulty in passing a motion, which sometimes appears to have the consistency of toothpaste, or the dog may become totally constipated. This benign enlargement of the prostate is cured by desexing but there are some cases where there is a malignancy in the prostate gland and this is naturally much more serious.

As a general rule, desex a female at about 6–7 months old or three months after her first season, and desex the male if he is making your life a misery but not until he is over 12 months of age.

# 14

# Body Language: Understanding Dogspeak

The art of 'reading' body language has become the 'in thing' over the past few years. People are at last waking up to the idea that the power of speech can in fact disguise what we are feeling and thinking rather than express it. Speech is of course sometimes used deliberately as a cover-up, but the fact is that no matter how articulate we may be, it is seldom that we can convey exactly what we have in our minds because our thoughts fly by far too quickly to be efficiently converted into speech. Our bodies often express the hidden or unarticulated contents of our minds.

Big business soon caught onto the art of interpreting and using body language with potential executives being taught how to 'read' the body language of the intimidating interviewer or to effectively disguise their own body's reaction in such a situation. How we humans complicate our lives!

Dogs are much more simple. Body language is a major part of their natural communication. But even they, no doubt because of their long association with humans, can use body language to con you! Your new puppy will soon develop this fine art to perfection. So here are a few pointers to interpreting your dog's body language so you have some idea of its intentions!

# A VOCABULARY OF DOGSPEAK

## Submissive urination

Puppies often throw themselves on their backs when they think you are cross with them. This is how a young pup in a pack, after it has stepped out of line, indicates to the pack leader that it has acknowledged them as the boss. The origin of the behaviour goes back even earlier than this. When the pup is suckling on its mother, she will roll it on its back once feeding is over, for a spit and polish. This treatment stimulates the pup to urinate and defecate; the mother then cleans it up.

Because you the owner have become the pup's replacement mother, the pup will slip into this conditioned reflex at the drop of a hat, especially if it is a pup with passive defence reflexes. All this means is that a pup is oversensitive to any signs of dominance in an owner, which can be as simple as looking menacingly tall. Such a reaction can also happen if you come home and the pup is overjoyed to see you in a mutually enthusiastic greeting; it then rolls onto its back and piddles all over its own tummy. Of course you are not about to get down on your knees and do what mother did to clean up the mess! But do be tolerant! Some owners, not realising the origin of this behaviour, will interpret it as a sign of the pup being dirty and not properly house-trained. But this behaviour has no connection with that. The pup is totally unaware of what it is doing and any show of displeasure on your part will only make the situation worse. Luckily the reflex to defecate at the same time leaves once solid food is introduced to the diet.

In order to train a pup out of this habit, an owner should follow a few simple rules. He or she should have a happy attitude when calling the pup, and should crouch down so as not to appear menacingly tall, looming over the pup. The owner should also put it in the sitting position when it comes to him and rub it on the front of the chest as a greeting – not a pat on the head, which is a dominant gesture. The pup soon becomes conditioned to 'recall' and 'sit' commands and as soon as the automatic throwing-itself-on-the-back reflex is broken, the pup stops this piddling habit.

## Licking

In the eyes of some owners, a dog licking is seen as the equivalent of kissing. In the eyes of other owners, however, with a pup who has licked itself on the backside and then tries to lick the owner on the face, the idea of doggy licking is, to put it mildly, highly distasteful!

What does licking mean in doggy language? It is mostly a genuine expression of affection but it is also closely linked to seeking attention, relieving tension and is sometimes used as a gesture to assert dominance.

Some owners are quite happy to let such behaviour go on, especially if it is satisfying to their egos. I would suggest, however, that you maintain regular worming so that licking does not become a health hazard. If you want to train a pup out of licking, simple obedience training usually does the trick and a consistent approach to this disciplining will normally train a dominant dog out of the habit. Should the cause of incessant licking be tension, the reason for the tension can usually be found with some careful thought and the problem addressed.

### Submissive and dominant – oldest tricks in the book

Dogs are capable of using both submissive and dominant behaviour to get their own way. This is where a dog's mastery of 'conning' an owner comes in. The placing of a paw on the master's lap is not a dog's way of trying to 'shake hands'. It is a deliberate attention-getting gesture to make you pat or play with it. This type of dog will also head-butt, lick or place its head on your lap to get your attention. It will even insidiously worm its way right into your lap if you let it. Your dog will then have effectively taught you to perform on command – you might well ask who is training who?

This same type of dog can also, of course, deliver a submissive message to get its own way: it can roll on its back with its legs in

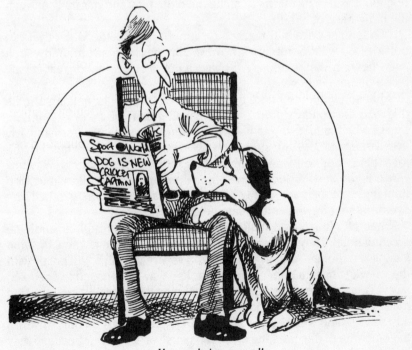

*You are being conned!*

the air, hopefully without the performance of submissive urination.

A dog would do this particular trick especially if you are angry about something, and it takes a very tough owner who can ignore such apologetic contrition! (Mind you, if you are the type of person who has not noticed how heart-wrenching this performance is, you might well be the type who has also not noticed many other of your dog's needs. But then of course you would probably not be reading this book!) There is nothing wrong in being 'conned' in this way for it's all part of the joys of dog ownership.

## Body language dog-to-dog
Although this situation will not apply to your young puppy, it is just as well to know early on how to read body language between adult dogs so that you can rid yourself of much of the anxiety and even fear that your pup may be attacked when you go out for a walk.

It is extremely rare for a dog to attack a pup. It simply isn't in the canine rules of playing the game. The only circumstances under which it could happen is if there is a genuine rogue dog on the loose. Such a dog is not a normal social animal, rather like a criminal in the human world. Often older dogs may turn on a pup and snarl but this is intended just to put the pup in its place because it has been pestering the older dog too much in its efforts to make the oldie play and naturally enough the oldie has got fed up.

Two female dogs will rarely have a right royal battle when they are outside for a walk. Sometimes, however, bitches in close proximity, such as living in the same house, will have a fierce confrontation, especially if one of them is in season.

What some people find particularly nerve-racking is walking a male dog who is strongly dominant. Recognising that you have a dominant pup can be the first step to help you control the situation from an early age. Dominant dogs are strongly territorial. When you walk them to the local park, they will want to mark their territory by urinating every few yards. If you keep a dog leashed, however, and do not allow it to stop until it gets to the park, you will reduce its natural tendency to become overdominant in your immediate neighbourhood.

When two unleashed male dogs meet, they go through an intricate greeting ritual. They sniff each other around the anal area where the anal glands are situated, and they may stand very rigid with a stiff tail or with the tail wagging in a rather tight, controlled way as opposed to a relaxed sway. Their hackles may rise and sometimes the dogs will growl. A dog may even mount another dog to show its dominance. Owners are best advised to stand well back as any gesture on their part can only mess up the outcome of this meeting and even cause an open war because they have accidentally reinforced the dominant feelings of their own dogs.

Once they have decided who is 'top dog' in the way known only to dogs, two males will usually turn away from each other and go and urinate on a post or tree. One dog may actually urinate on top of where the other has marked. Once this ritual has been gone through uninterrupted there is usually no cause for further worry.

If a dog is in an area with which it is familiar, it is much more likely to adopt the dominant position. If two dogs of equal dominance meet therefore, a fight is likely to ensue. Sometimes if you keep your cool and do not interfere, the fight will be over in a minute and the top dog position will have been established for the time being at least. Then is the owners' chance to leash their dogs and go their separate ways. Once the dogs are out of each other's territory, they will not head for each other again when taken off leash.

If a serious fight does break out, having a hose handy is a good 'fight-stopper'. But of course this is unlikely out on a walk. Instead, grasp the dog by the testicles and slightly twist them; this is very effective. If, as an empathetic male owner, you cannot twist testicles, a twist of the flank skin also works. The two owners need to do this at the same time to stop the fight fair and square. Dogs, like people, either have a rapport, openly dislike each other or are totally indifferent. They do initiate friendships with other dogs. A dog will invite another dog to play by bouncing

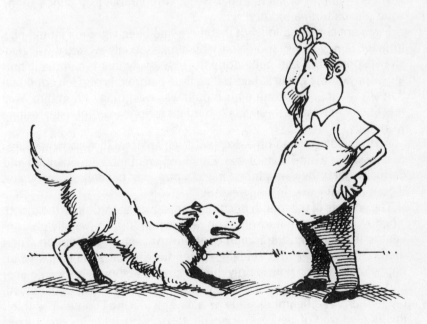

*A play invitation.*

low on the front legs with its rear end up in the air. Your dog will do the same performance with you and you can instigate play by making some sort of imitative gesture like bounding on your feet and bobbing your head down.

**Stress behaviour**
Your pup's or dog's body language may be expressing stress. If a family are having a screaming match, yelling at each other or throwing things, a dog can react in a stressed manner by destructive behaviour. This behaviour may be directed at itself such as in chewing lumps off its front legs, chewing the pads on its feet, or overgrooming its feet. If your dog is acting like this, maybe you are in need of some family counselling!

**Facial expressions: do dogs smile?**
You can tell a great deal about a pup from the expressions on its face as well as those on the face of an adult dog. Once, a 7-week-old pup came to the surgery for its vaccinations. As usual I was watching carefully for any signs that would tell me if the owners were going about things the wrong way. Sure enough, as I went to look at the puppy's teeth and tonsils, the pup growled and actually drew back the corners of its mouth, curling the lips right up. This was an overly dominant gesture from one of such tender years, comparable to a punch in the solar plexus from a toddler!

I was not surprised to learn that there had been vigorous mouth-play from the family's 10-year-old son, which had not only evoked the aggressive response but had been done in such a way that it had really hurt the puppy. It was going to take a long time before this pup felt confident that any attempt to examine his mouth was not going to hurt him. This reaction of fear made it especially hard for anyone to administer routine wormings.

A wrinkled forehead on a dog indicates anxiety. Showing the whites of the eyes is a sure sign of fear. Ears held erect indicate attention and curiosity but if they are pinned back, a pup may be feeling anxious or, if coupled with snarling, aggressive.

The corners of the mouth position themselves according to the mood. 'Slightly up' denotes relaxed happiness while 'drawn back' with concentric lines around the mouth often means pain or discomfort. Then there are the dogs who actually smile, drawing back their lips when happy and greeting you. Mainly this is done in response to people only and I believe it is evidence of an imitative ability. 'Outsiders', of course, often interpret a beaming smile as a savage affront. I sometimes think this is also true of people, especially those whose smiles are a fixed grimace with no smiling twinkle in the eye!

## Long-distance communication

Consider the following scene. You are in the park walking your dog and another dog appears on the horizon. 'Is this going to mean trouble?' you wonder. The other dog is looking your way, standing stock still. Your dog has seen it and is also like a frozen statue. Then suddenly one dog drops down to the lying position. Everyone can breathe a sigh of relief as there is not going to be a confrontation. The dog who has dropped to the lying position has assumed the submissive role and thereby acknowledged the other dog as being the dominant one. The dogs in this situation may be two males, a male and a female, or two females. Whatever the combination, it takes a dog to make a decision like that long distance! As a friend once said to me about people: 'You can't see a beautiful mind across a crowded room!'

Males and females seldom fight, although females are often very stroppy in their attitude to male dogs, especially if he shows an interest in her and she is not inclined to reciprocate. She can snap at him and nip him but it is almost unheard of for a male dog to retaliate. He lowers the head in a submissive gesture and turns away, always the perfect gentleman!

# 15

# Training

## WHY BOTHER?

When you go to training classes with your dog, you teach it to sit, to go down into the lying position, to stay in one spot until you call it and to walk neatly at your side (called walking to heel). Now, you may say, why bother? Like Mr Barton who said he didn't give a damn if his dog stood up or sat down while waiting for him outside the bottle shop as long as he didn't wander off! Then there was Miss Barlow who declared she did not want her dog bossed around by her; she wanted it to be a friend, on an equal footing, so to speak.

Now, what Mr Barton did not understand was that unless his dog was put through this routine training until the lessons were thoroughly consolidated, he would not have a hope of trusting his dog not to wander off. As for Miss Barlow, if she continued her attitude, she would end up with a thoroughly indulged dog who did precisely as it liked and not, as she anthropomorphised, by discussing things with her first! It would just have 'pack-leadered' her!

The object of training is to fit the pup into the family situation with the minimum of fuss. By going through this routine training, the dog learns to respect you as pack leader. If it has any problems in its behaviour, you cannot hope to modify these in an untrained dog. In fact, once a dog starts training, behaviour problems often miraculously disappear because you have become boss. The dog knows where it is and does not indulge in delinquency because it feels secure in the more intimate and secure relationship it is getting from you.

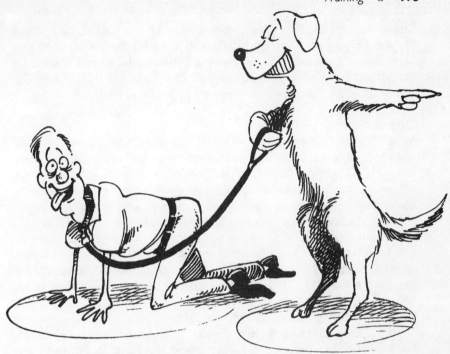

*Without routine training your dog may pack-leader you.*

Also, training extends the dog's world of experience beyond the backyard, which is far too narrow an existence, to the outside world where you can help develop the dog's confidence in the face of all sorts of threats. Just the right balance is needed. A nervous dog, displaying submissive tendencies before training, needs a special approach, while a dog trained with too much heavy compulsion could easily become far too suppressed and submissive.

# TRAINING METHODS

Now that your pup is 6 months old it is of age to attend formal training classes. On the other hand, you may decide to have a go yourself.

### By the book
There are many good training manuals on the market but check when a book was first published as training methods have changed radically over the years. For example, compulsive methods have long gone out of date and physical punishment is never necessary. Also be aware that some books have been republished but the teaching material has not been properly updated.

Often different types of dogs and different types of people need totally different methods of training. You may read a book, find nothing works for you or your dog and get thoroughly disillusioned. Where do you seek ongoing advice? This is where a professional trainer should be consulted. For a start, however, get as many training books from the library as you can and see how you go by trial and error.

### Dog clubs

Most cities of the world have dog-training classes that meet regularly at a local park and train dogs to a varying standard of obedience. Joining such clubs is not limited to pedigree dogs. Some dogs and owners achieve a very high standard in these classes and end up entering obedience training, tracking and agility trials as well as dog shows.

It is also excellent for your pup to have the experience of mixing with all the other dogs at these clubs, but in the early days at least, classes can be a hilarious circus. Some dogs leap up and deposit wet kisses on their owners' faces, roll on their backs or refuse to move, while a few have a total nervous breakdown and collapse in a shivering heap. Some dogs want to tear all the others apart while others behave like Goody-Two-Shoes and do everything right.

This clearly indicates the drawbacks of 'all-breeds' training classes. Each dog needs a different training method and being in a mixed class can limit the success of some of the participants. Also, dogs are not brilliant at concentrating for long. As the classes only meet about once a week and the conscientious dog owner is certainly not going to attend for just a quarter of an hour, this means that many dogs get fed up after a while in these long classes and start to play up.

A young dog can also be overtrained. I remember a patient, a highly intelligent German shepherd dog, who demonstrated training classes on a television programme with his owner and a trainer. The demands of constant performance imposed a great deal of strain on the dog who later developed problems of aggression.

Many people who join such classes drop out disillusioned and this is because class sizes are such that a trainer cannot possibly give attention to all the handlers and all the dogs. So, if you fall into this disillusioned category after attending a number of classes, do not give up on either your dog or yourself. You may well have a dog who is potentially brilliant – just like those children who refuse to learn at school and then, after they drop out, later become self-made millionaires! Dogs are often boisterous, inattentive or aggressive (anyone recognise a description of their dog or child?) but when working on a one-to-one basis they can turn out to be brilliant. Unfortunately, some bright dogs are left to languish in the hands of an owner who is slow to catch on with training methods.

Much depends on the temperament of the dog. A dog may feel threatened by the close proximity of so many other dogs and this means it will not be able to concentrate. As a result, the handler will lose control and confidence. It is hard for even a professional handler to get any success with a dog who is thoroughly distracted. Of course the ultimate aim is to have a dog totally obedient in the face of all tempting distractions but sometimes this kind of concentration has to come later.

There are owners who get embarrassed by the antics of their 'little darlings' at training classes. Others resent authority to the extent that they even find it hard to accept a handler issuing positive instructions while extremely shy people cannot cope with the public pressure of a class situation. For a learner, handling a dog is just like starting to drive a car or operating a new piece of computer hardware. It feels awkward at first and it takes practice to develop a relaxed manner and work with style, co-ordinating leash technique with verbal commands.

If you are not excessively shy and do not worry what people think of you, and you have a dog with a stable temperament and no behavioural problems, then all-breeds training classes should work very well for you. They are also cheap to attend. It is wise to go along for a couple of weekends and just be an observer without your dog. This way you can assess class sizes and results as clubs do vary in their efficiency.

### Training kennels
The Ladbrooks were a very busy family so they opted to send their young dog to a kennel for a month to be trained. When they went to pick him up, the trainer demonstrated the results of his work. They were most impressed. Off they went home and out into the garden to put Barnaby through his paces. He sat obediently for a split second and then leapt up and bounded about behaving in his usual larrikin way! The experience of the trainer and his quiet intimidation of Barnaby made the training results look spectacular but, away from this situation, the dog simply reverted to his old ways. This was a very expensive lesson and is a very common story!

A common claim by some trainers is the success of the six-minute method. Most handlers can make a dog look 'trained' almost instantly to the uneducated by utilising good handling technique, quiet intimidation and working close to the dog. In fact, many owners report that the trainer has appeared to hypnotise their dog! Of course, it is a total illusion that the dog has been 'trained', because as soon as it is handed back to the owner, it carries on just as it did before. A correctly trained dog means that it will obey commands at all times, especially off leash.

You have to have your wits about you if you are going to avail yourself of this most common method of dog training. Not only is it the most lucrative for the trainer, it is the most abused by them. You have no idea how many dogs are booked into the kennels at a time, so of course you have no clue as to whether your dog did have lessons on a regular basis during its stay. A five-week period of training is probably best as a dog has to adjust to its new temporary environment and learn to socialise with other dogs.

So how can you check that you are not being taken for a ride? You should visit the kennel, talk to the trainer and ask to see some dogs at varying stages undergoing training. Kennels often demonstrate with dogs at the completion of their training, but if you can see dogs at different stages then you have a better idea as to the success of the kennels' methods. It is also essential to watch a dog in off-leash work, to properly assess the results. Unless the dog is old, has a well-entrenched behavioural problem or is neurotic, an off-leash standard of training should be attained. Be very wary of the trainer who guarantees results. This is just not possible until a profile has been done on dog, owner and environment. Comparison of a few training kennels stands you in good stead. Also ask around to see what other people's experiences have been like.

If dogs come home smelling like a sewage plant or are unduly skinny, forget the place. You must be convinced that your dog is going to be *cared for*. For this you have to trust to your own instincts. Can cruelty be a factor? Unfortunately it can. Some trainers use heavy compulsion on every dog.

### Home training
Having a professional trainer come to the home can be ideal if the owner is shy or self-conscious at communal classes or does not want their dog boarded while training. It can in fact sort out a dog with problems.

What can you expect from this type of training? At least six lessons of an hour to an hour and a half, once a week, are necessary for good results. The first lesson is mainly an assessment of the dog's temperament and gives the trainer a good indication of the home environment of the dog, to say nothing of the owner! The dog's habits should be recorded and any problems that are beginning to show up should be discussed. This should be followed up by a crash-course in dog psychology, highlighting the objects to be achieved in the course of the training.

The dog and owner are then trained through a series of exercises that the owner practises through the rest of the week. Now this is where the process can come badly unstuck if the owner does not practise daily for short but fairly frequent intervals. If you have not consolidated the training in the first week, then you cannot expect any progress the following week, and will have to go over old ground. Any interruptions such as wet weather or sickness can seriously jeopardise the system.

Meeting other members of the family can help the trainer see where behavioural problems might be originating. Training is initially carried out in the dog's own immediate environment but progresses to outside areas such as local parks, streets, shopping centres, noisy railway stations and, in fact, anywhere there are distractions that the dog must learn to ignore. This is essential as controlling a dog in a difficult situation is a must. For example, you have come home from work and your dog is just coming out of the front gate with another member of the family. The dog is off leash, something you have never worried about because you live in a quiet area. The dog sees you and makes a wild dash to welcome you but he does not make it. A car kills him outright. If his obedience training had been up to scratch, then you could have made him stay where he was until the danger had passed.

### Attack-trained dogs
In a world sadly dominated by greed and drugs, security in the home has become top priority, especially among those who regard material possessions as a life goal. This obsession with security has created a demand for attack-trained dogs. We cannot stress enough what a disastrous trend this is. Statistics show that the correctly trained dog hardly ever needs to actually attack. Its presence is deterrent enough. Any territorially minded dog can fulfil the same function.

Many so-called attack-trained dogs are not trained correctly and their presence, especially in a normal household, can be a real danger to members of its own human family as well as innocent visitors and passers by. Even with non-attack-trained dogs, there have been tragedies of maulings, and even death of young children who were playing happily with a bunch of young dogs. Because the child's reaction is not like that of a litter mate, it all goes horribly wrong as sibling aggression in the adolescent dogs towards the child has gone overboard, resulting in a bad bite, and even death.

# Epilogue

If you have used this book for rearing pups correctly, let's hope you will have many happy years with your dog as a companion. The time will come when it reverts to some aspects of puppyhood, like not coming when you call it and having toilet accidents in the house. There is nothing you can do to train it this time. It is due to the sadness of old age when the messages from the brain get scrambled up. Once again, you need loving patience to put up with a now geriatric friend in senility, going through a second puppyhood. But that is another story.

# Index

affenpinscher 28
Afghan hound 15, 48, 105
Airedale terrier 35
akita 61–2
Alaskan malamute 62
allergies 94, 124, 129, 144, 145, 146
Alsatian *see* German shepherd dog
American cocker spaniel 45
American foxhound 51
American Staffordshire terrier 35
American water spaniel 46
Anatolian shepherd 54–5
antibiotics 115, 116, 118, 161
arthritis 20, 69
attack-trained dogs 177
Australian cattle dog 55
Australian kelpie 55–6
Australian silky terrier 28
Australian terrier 35–6

baby-talk 113
back problems 50
basenji 48
basset hound 20, 48–9, 123
bathing 15, 120–2, 143, 145
beagle 47, 49, 128
bearded collie 59–60
bedding 144

Bedlington terrier 36
behavioural problems 16, 24–5, 76–7, 78, 96
Belgian shepherd 56
Bernese mountain dog 62
bichon frise 29
biting 17, 82, 103, 155
black and tan coon hound 49
bloodhound 50
bobtail 58
body language (dog) 98, 165–71
bone malformations 20, 66, 94
bones 94
border collie 54, 59, 60
border terrier 36
boredom 40, 81, 94, 132
borzoi 50
Boston terrier 67, 128
Bouvier des Flandres 56
boxer 62
brabancon 31
breathing problems 20, 33, 67, 71
breed clubs 22
breed development 19–20
breed guide 27–72
breeders 20–4, 71
breeders' diets 87

brewer's yeast 146
Briard 56
British bulldog 20, 67, 128
Brittany spaniel 45
brushing 120–1
bulky stools 90
bull terrier 36
  miniature 36
bullmastiff 63
butterfly dog 32

cairn terrier 36–7
calcium 90, 93
cancer 40, 85, 160, 164
canned food 87, 88–91
Cardigan corgi 61
carsickness 76
Cavalier King Charles spaniel 29
chain-lead 99
Chesapeake Bay retriever 42, 128
chihuahua 29–30
children and dogs 3–4
Chinese crested dog 30
Chinese fighting dog 71
choke-chain 99, 107
choosing a dog 3–25
chorea 116
chow chow 68, 128
claws 65, 122, 132

cleaning up after dog 9
clipping 70, 148
clumber spaniel 45
cocker spaniel 45–6, 132
collar 103, 155, 156
collie 21, 59–61
confinement 76–7, 78, 83–4,
    101–2
constipation 164
contraceptive pill 161
coprophagia 84–5
corgi 21, 131–2
cosmetic surgery 130–2
cough medicine 118
country tapeworm 136,
    137–8
couples and dogs 4–5
crossbreeds 18, 55–6
curly-coated retriever 42

dachshund 48, 50
Dalmatian 68
Dandie Dinmont terrier 37
deafness 68
debarking 132
deerhound 51
defaecation 9, 23, 80–1,
    84–5, 90, 131, 164
demodectic mange 148–9
desexing 13, 16, 121, 156,
    157–64
dew claws 65, 122, 132
diabetes 50
diet alternatives 91–3
diet quantities 87–8
diet requirements 88–91,
    94–5
diet supplements 91, 93–4
diet taboos 94
*Dipylidium caninum* 136–7
discipline 76, 98, 102–4,
    106–8
dislocated lenses 37
distemper 114, 115–16, 119
Dobermann 63
dog clubs 174–5
dog coats 15, 30, 31
dog-tag 155
dog-to-dog body language
    100, 168–70, 171
dominant behaviour 82, 93,
    166, 167, 170
dosing 129–30, 131
dried food 87, 89
Dutch barge dog 69

ear care 123–6
ear cropping 132

ear problems 12, 45, 46,
    123–6
eardrops 123–4, 126
*Echinococcus granulosus*
    136, 137–8
elderly and dogs 5–7
elkhound 54
English foxhound 51
English setter 44
English Staffordshire bull
    terrier 35
English toy spaniel 29
English toy terrier 30–1
epilepsy 20, 69
eucalyptus oil 146
external parasites 140–9
eye care 33, 128–9
eye problems 12, 20, 37, 45,
    61
eyelid problems 20, 71, 128

face problems 68, 128
facial expressions 170
false pregnancy 160
fear biter 17, 24–5, 155
fear imprinting 17, 85–6, 99
feeding *see* diet
female dogs 12
    desexing 157–9
    undesexed 159–61
fennel seed 146
field spaniel 45
fights 169, 171
Finnish spitz 54
flat-coated retriever 42
flea allergy 146
flea collar 142–3, 145
flea powder 146
fleas 121, 137, 140–6
food allergies 94
fox terrier
    smooth 37
    wire 37
French bulldog 68
fussy eaters 89

games 81–3, 102–4
garlic 86, 146
gazelle hound 53
German pinscher 63
German shepherd dog 56–7
German short-haired pointer
    41
German spitz 69
German wire-haired pointer
    42
*Giardia* 139
glaucoma 37

Glen of Imaal terrier 37
goitre 37
golden retriever 43, 128
Gordon setter 44
grass seeds 124
grass tick 147-8
Great Dane 69, 128
greyhound 41, 51–2, 130–1
griffon a poli laineux 22
griffon Bruxellois 31
gun dogs 40–7

haemophilia 20
hair-conditioner 15, 121
halters 108
Hamiltonstovare 52
hand-feeding 90
hard pad 116
harrier 51
health care 111–49
health guarantee 16, 17
healthy pup 11–12
heartworm 139–40
heeler 55
hepatitis 116–17, 119
hernias 131
hiccoughs 88
hip dysplasia 20, 57, 58, 94
home training 176–7
hookworm 135–6
hormone replacement
    therapy 159
hounds 47–54
house training 23, 77, 78–9,
    80–1
Hungarian puli 20, 57
Hungarian vizsla 46
hydatid disease 136, 137–8
hyperactivity 3, 83

Ibizan hound 52
identification 155–6
immune system problems
    71, 88, 149
immunity 116
in season 158, 159–60, 168
inherited problems 37, 45,
    53, 61, 68, 69, 71, 94, 128
insect growth hormone
    inhibitor 143, 144–5
insecticides 141, 142–4, 148,
    149
insurance 153–6
internal parasites 133–40
Irish red and white setter 44
Irish setter 44, 128
Irish terrier 37
Irish water spaniel 46

Irish wolfhound 14, 52
isolation stress 47
Italian greyhound 31
Italian spinone 46–7
*Ixodes holocyclus* 147–8

Jack Russell terrier 37–8
Japanese chin 31
Japanese spaniel 31
Japanese spitz 69

kangaroo meat 94
karabash 54–5
keeshond 69
kennel 78
kennel cough 117–18
Kerry blue 38
kidney stones 68
King Charles spaniel 29
komondor 63
Kuvasz 57–8

Labrador retriever 14, 40, 43,
    105
Lakeland terrier 38
large dogs 14, 15, 162–3
late-maturing breeds 105
leads 99, 106
leg problems 12, 49, 66
Leonberger 63
leptospirosis 117
lick granuloma 40, 85
licking 166–7
lion dog 33
llasa apso 69–70
loneliness 83–5
lowchen 31
lying down command 108,
    172

male dogs 12–13
Maltese 32
mammary cancer 160
Manchester terrier 30, 38
    toy 30–1
mange 148–9
Maremma sheepdog 58
market places 17
marking 12–13, 162, 168,
    169
mastiff 19, 34, 64, 67
medicine 129–30, 131
methylated spirit 146
Mexican hairless dog 32
microchip identification 155
milk allergy 94
miniature pinscher 32
mites 124

mongrel *see* crossbreed
mosquito 139–40
mouth infections 46, 128
mouth-shy 126–7, 171
Munsterlander (large) 47

nails 65, 122–3, 132
natural diet 90–1
Neopolitan mastiff 64
Newfoundland 64–5
night blindness 20
non-sporting dogs 67–72
Norfolk terrier 38
Norwegian buhund 58
Norwich terrier 38
Nova Scotia duck-tolling
    retriever 43–4
nursing 83, 167
nutrition 87–95

oatmeal soap 146
obedience training 99
offal 137, 138
Old English sheepdog 58,
    105
oral insecticides 143–4
otterhound 52
outcrossing 42
overdependence 75, 76, 83
oversexed dogs 162, 163

pack-leader 5, 8, 24, 25, 30,
    68, 97, 105, 172
papillon 32
parasites 133–49
Parson Jack Russell terrier
    38
parvovirus 116, 117, 119
patting 76, 166
pedicure 122–3
pedigree dogs 14, 18–25,
    27–8
Pekingese 20, 33, 128, 129
Pembroke corgi 61
pen 77, 78, 83–4, 102
personal territory 106
pet shops 17
Petit Basset Griffon
    Vendeen 53
Pharaoh hound 52
Phu Quoc 53
pit bull terrier 35
pit dog 35
playing 81–3, 102–4, 169–70
plum pudding dog *see*
    Dalmatian
pointers 41–2
Polish lowland sheepdog 58

Pomeranian 33
poodle 70, 129
Portuguese water dog 65
post-distemper encephalitis
    114, 115–16
pounds 15–17
praising 76, 80, 101
pregnancy 134–5
primitive dogs 18–19, 20
prostate problems 164
pug 33–4
pumi 58
punishment 80, 102, 106
pup selection test 18, 25–6
purchasing a pup 11–26
pyometra 160–1
Pyrenean mountain dog 65,
    132
pyrethrum insecticide 143,
    144

rabies 118–19
raw meat 90, 91
recall training 101, 106
registration 156
rest 83
retinal atrophy 20, 61
retrievers 42–4
Rhodesian ridgeback 53
ringworm 149
roaming 99, 100
Rottweiler 65
rough collie 60
rough play 103
roundworm 133–5, 136
routines 84, 102
ruffle pups *see* shar-pei

St Bernard 66, 128
saluki 53
Samoyed 66, 130
sarcoptic mange 149
scabies 149
schipperke 71
schnauzer 66, 132
Scottish terrier 40
Sealyham terrier 38–9
seed tick 147–8
selecting from litter 24–6
self-mutilation 85
separation anxiety 16, 47,
    78, 83–4
setters 44
sexual maturity 100, 105
shampoo 15, 121, 143, 145
shar-pei 71
sheltie 59
Shetland sheepdog 59

shiba inu 66
shih tzu 71
Siberian husky 62, 66–7
sit command 108, 172
skin care 30, 146
skin problems 40, 61, 68, 71, 85, 88, 146
Skye terrier 39
sleeping arrangements 77–80
sleeve dog *see* Pekingese
sloughi 53–4
smalandsstovare 22
small dogs 13–14, 161–2
smooth collie 60–1
soft-coated wheaten terrier 39
spaniel 20, 45–6, 128
*Spirometra erinacei* 138
spitz dogs 28, 33, 54, 58, 62, 66, 68, 69, 71
springer spaniel 45–6
squirrel spaniel 32
Staffordshire bull terrier 39
status-symbol dogs 8, 69
stealing food 93
stress 16, 47, 62, 78, 83–4, 85, 96, 170
stumpy-tailed cattle dog 59
subcutaneous injection 112
submissive behaviour 166, 167–8
submissive urination 166

Sussex spaniel 46
Swedish vallhund 59

tablets 129–30
*Taenia hydatigena* 138
*Taenia ovis* 138
tail docking 58, 130–2
tapeworm 136–40, 141
tea-tree oil 146
teething 126
terriers 34–40
territory 12–13, 100, 162–3, 168, 169
testicular cancer 164
third eyelid 128–9
Tibetan mastiff 67
Tibetan spaniel 72
Tibetan terrier 71–2
tick collar 148
tick poisoning 147–8
ticks 146–8
Timmins' biter *see* stumpy-tailed cattle dog
titbits 92–3
tooth care 126–8
tooth problems 28
town tapeworm 136–7, 141
toy dogs 28–34
toys 81
training 49, 98, 172–7
training kennels 175
training manuals 173–4
travelling with puppy 75–6

ultrasonic collar 143
undesexed bitch 158, 159–61
undesexed male 161–3
urinating 12–13, 23, 76, 77, 78–9, 80–1, 162, 168, 169
utility dogs 61–7

vaccination 16, 99, 111–12, 114–19, 121
vegan diet 91
vegetarian diet 91
visiting the vet 111–13
vitamins 88, 93–4

walking 9–10, 99, 101
walking to heel 107–8, 172
warts 146
wax (ear) 123, 126
Weimaraner 47
Welsh corgi 61
Welsh springer 46
Welsh terrier 39–40
West Highland white terrier 40
wetterhund 22
whippet 54
whipworm 136
working dogs 54–61
worms 84, 87, 88, 133–40

Yorkshire terrier 34
young singles and dogs 7–8